Beautiful from Within

THE SURPRISING POWER OF NUTRITION

FOR

HAIR, SKIN, AND NAILS

D. Lewis

Author
D. Lewis

docdawa@gmail.com

Graphics and Book Layout
Peter Brooks Hale

ISBN-13: 978-1508526100

ISBN-10: 1508526109

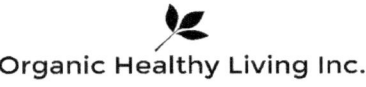

Organic Healthy Living Inc.
Publications
2015
Fort Collins, Colorado

Beautiful from Within

You are what you eat."

"You are only as pretty as you feel."

"Beauty is not just skin deep...
Beauty comes from within."

Table of Contents

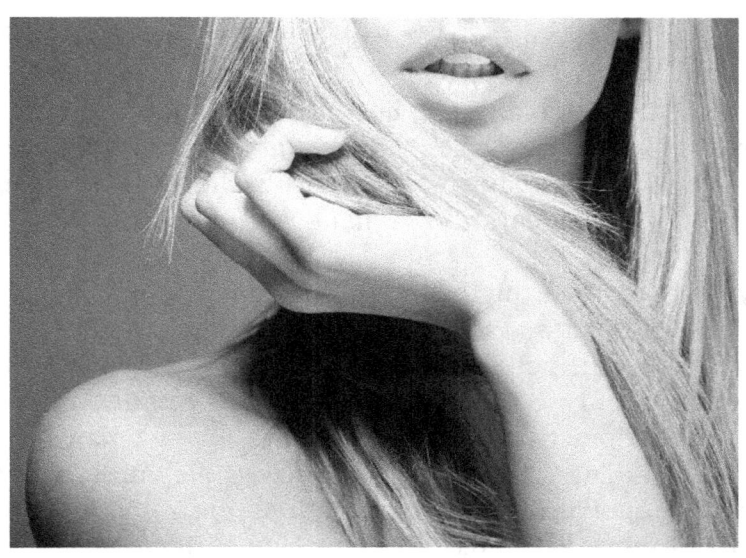

Beautiful from Within

Introduction

You are what you eat." "You are only as pretty as you feel." "Beauty is not just skin deep… beauty comes from within." These three simple statements sum up the philosophy behind *Beautiful from Within: The Surprising Power of Nutrition for Hair, Skin, and Nails.*

Our hair, skin, and nails— indeed, all of our bodily tissues— are made from the molecules in the food we ingest. This is the most basic rule in nutrition: we are what we eat. As I always tell my students, the obvious conclusion to this statement is "if we eat junk food, then we will have a junky body." By the same token, if we eat healthy, nourishing, beautiful food, we will have a healthy, well-nourished body that looks its best.

Beautiful from Within: *The Surprising Power of Nutrition for Hair, Skin, and Nails* is every woman's user's manual for optimal nourishment for looking her best. Our hair, skin, and nails are the external reflection of the inner state of the body; knowing how and what nourishes each tissue is the key to having the healthy, vibrant appearance we all desire.

In my years of lecturing to cosmetology and esthetician students and their instructors, as well as to broader audiences, I have constantly reaffirmed that "nutrition is not rocket science." Neither is it boring, irrelevant science. *Beautiful from Within* brings nutrition to the forefront of any woman's beauty program, making it simple, fun, accessible, and above all, relevant. Empowering women to adopt the nutritional know-how to optimize their looks is the mission of Beauty from Within. Lustrous, healthy hair; firmer, more elastic skin; and strong nails can all be obtained through following the simple protocols and recommendations contained in *Beautiful from Within*.

Beautiful from Within specifies which nutrients are best for what tissues. But *Beautiful from Within* does not merely recommend endless bottles of vitamins and minerals. A key message of *Beautiful from Within* is that food is still our appearance's best friend. As it turns out, foods that are considered "nutrient-dense" (or "nude") sources of key nutrients are easily adopted as "beauty foods." A nutrient-dense diet is the best way to ensure maximum health, vitality, and beauty.

Encouraging, empowering, and supporting women to reacquaint themselves with the pleasures and gratification of shopping, cooking, and preparing "real" food is another important aspect of *Beautiful from Within*. So much of our modern life is about shortcuts and quick fixes. Yet most women know intuitively that quick fixes and shortcuts are probably not the easiest or best ways to go about creating, building, and maintaining one's looks for the long run.

We do only look as pretty as we feel, and real food is one of the most important foundations we have for feeling our best. Real health takes time and work to maintain and sustain. Eating well is sometimes simply about reacquainting ourselves with the basics. Eating a diet of mostly junk and fast food may be convenient, but it probably won't help us achieve our long-term health and beauty goals.

Beauty and health go hand in hand. In talking to students, I frequently remind them that "you are only as pretty as you feel." I illustrate this by pointing out that you won't look your best if you are walking around with a scowl on your face from a headache or if you are slumped over from stress or a stomachache. Health, vibrant energy, confidence, enthusiasm, and a positive outlook are all also important parts of the message of *Beautiful from Within.*

To that end, this book affirms the importance of stress reduction, getting enough sleep, exercise, time out for oneself, fresh air and deep breathing, a positive outlook and, of course, drinking enough pure water for hydration. Encouraging a proactive, can-do stance, *Beautiful from Within* provides the important role of being a supportive cheerleader, information source, and mentor for today's active woman.

Beautiful from Within was born from lectures I have given to countless beauty/cosmetology/esthetician school students with an eye towards empowering them to better provide for their clients by giving them a knowledgeable nutritional edge. Virtually all women want to know what they can do— what they can eat or take— to improve the quality of their appearance, and cosmetologists and estheticians are in the perfect position to offer such advice. But the scope of *Beautiful from Within* is not limited to professionals; rather it is designed for all women who wish to take such advice into their own hands.

Beauty and health are perennially among the most important topics for women. A large percentage of women spend more on their appearance than virtually any other expenditure. Women crave the confidence that comes from knowing they look their best, yet too often feel unsure as to how to optimize their appearance. *Beautiful from Within* lets women know that good , credible information is available—information that is confidence boosting, accessible, and easy to implement.

One final thought: in today's fast-paced and ever-changing world, we sometimes can forget to take time out for ourselves. We need to remember to balance our own needs with the demands of our family, friends, and community. Love yourself— and treat your body and yourself with the dignity and respect you so richly deserve!

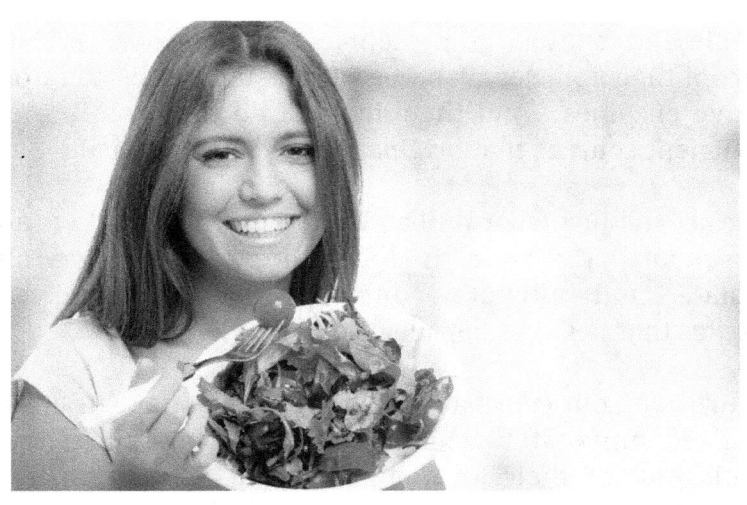

Chapter 1

You _Are_ What You Eat

"You are what you eat." This is the most fundamental lesson in nutrition. Every cell- indeed every molecule in your body- is made from the atoms and molecules that you eat, breathe, and drink. It turns out that your outer environment and your inner landscape are not all that different. What we ingest affects us- in ways both profound and subtle- and for better and for worst.

Our cells are constantly working, doing their best to sustain and maintain us- often despite our best attempts to undermine their mission! Cells must metabolize nutrients and deal with toxins and poisons in order to accomplish their often challenging tasks. Cells assemble and manufacture complex molecules such as hormones and other chemicals. They have to breathe, secrete, excrete, divide, and grow just like any organism. Hair cells must assemble and grow large proteinaceous molecules that we call hair from their follicles. Pancreatic cells must secrete important digestive enzymes. And they must all do this from the energy and nutrient sources that originate in the foods we eat.

But we are not just what we eat. We are literally what we absorb, or assimilate. Digestion is the process where we absorb, assimilate, and ultimately incorporate into ourselves the molecules that begin as our meals and snacks.

As it turns out, our cells have to put up with a lot. Cells are highly specialized units of biological complexity and integrity, and depending upon their location and need, can do an amazing array of things. Bone cells become ossified, calcified objects of support and strength, while a liver cell has entirely different metabolic functions and roles to play. Similarly, a cell that makes up part of your skin has different needs, roles, and stresses than a cell that secretes stomach acid from within the lining of your stomach. Nerve cells must transmit and receive chemical and electrical messages from other nerve cells. But all have the same basic requirements: the proper quality and quantity of nutrients to replace, replenish, and resupply what is used up during the cell's life.

The beauty tissues- our hair, skin, and nails- are no exception. In order to be their best, we need to supply them with all the necessary ingredients they require. And ideally we should try and protect them from too many of the wrong things- chemicals and other environmental factors- that challenge, damage, or stress them.

Optimizing your health- and your looks- is ultimately your responsibility, alone. We can go to trainers, fitness experts, doctors, or our favorite hair stylist- but ultimately, it is what we do as the inhabitants of our own bodies- the choices we make-that will determine if we age faster or slower, if we are fit or fat, if we remain healthy or fall ill. Of course, there are additional factors such as our genetics and the various environmental situations and exposures that we may have no control over, but in general we could say that our daily choices and actions have a *huge* role to play in how we feel- and look.

Because we are each faced with innumerable choices every day, we need to be as knowledgeable as possible. Today's world is so complex, and we are exposed to so many influences- many of which did not even exist a generation or two ago. No longer can we afford the luxury of saying "if I had only known", or "why didn't anyone tell me?" EMF radiation, cancer-causing chemicals, artificial food additives, man-made contaminants added to our drinking and bathing water, some prescription drugs, and harsh soaps or detergents are just some of the many things we may be confronted with today on a frighteningly consistent basis. Just as it is our personal choice whether or not to smoke cigarettes, it is also our personal choice whether or not we choose to invite in or keep certain chemicals and additives out of our bodies by selecting organic foods over conventional ones. Similarly, we may choose to install a shower or home filter to take skin and hair-drying chlorine out of our water. Of course there are countless other examples of what we invite into our world- from the brand of shampoo or soap we buy to getting a radiation-protective screen for our computer.

The point is, we are ultimately responsible for what goes on with our bodies, and our health. I admit that this can be daunting- even intimidating- but, really, there is little choice in the matter. And, this may even be ultimately empowering. We may not want to be experts at nutrition or holistic health, and we don't have to be- but we should at least have enough basic knowledge so that we feel competent to make somewhat informed choices. I think if you know enough to use your intuition and common sense, then that is a *great* start.

My basic rule of thumb is to "err on the side of caution". Because we are dealing with something as important as our very health, it simply doesn't make a lot of sense to gamble with it. Much in the modern world in general -and in the science of nutrition in particular- is controversial. Naturally those with vested interests and economic incentives will always defend their products and their safety. But if we look around us, we see alarming signs that our nutrition and health as a nation isn't all that it could be. Obesity, heart disease, cancer, diabetes, lack of energy, depression, and learning disabilities are all at unprecedented and epidemic levels. Perhaps we should ask ourselves if something is not quite right with this picture. America is a great country, yet we are suffering with an incredible array of health problems, right here, right now. We have a huge collective health problem, and an accompanying economic burden as well.

So, as an individual, you have the unique situation where you still get to call the shots! Food-how you nourish yourself- is one of the true freedoms we all still have available to us. What you choose to put into your mouth- and body- is ultimately your decision, alone. And knowing that you deserve the best is an important part of the "beautiful from within" philosophy.

Self-esteem, dignity, and self-respect are concepts that I feel strongly reflect the *BFW* view. Basically, how we view and feel about ourselves is vitally important to the choices we will make throughout our lives. If you strongly feel you deserve only the best because you expect nothing less than great health and the looks that go along with it, then you are likely going to do the things necessary to ensure that you stay healthy, such as exercising and eating right.

On the other hand, if you don't deeply feel you deserve great health, you are more likely to choose behaviors and patterns that will ultimately undermine your health. People who smoke or drink too much, and who eat poor quality junk foods, probably don't really feel that great health is attainable, or worth the effort- or perhaps that they even deserve it. They may feel that good health is out of their reach, and so don't really try to strive for it.

If you are serious about embarking upon the *"Beautiful from Within"* program, I encourage you to think deeply about these things. Great achievements are in reach for you, but only if you take them seriously enough to give them a real shot. Your life- your health, your looks, and your peace of mind- are in *your* hands. I strongly encourage you to think about your relationship with your food- and its intimate connection with your body.

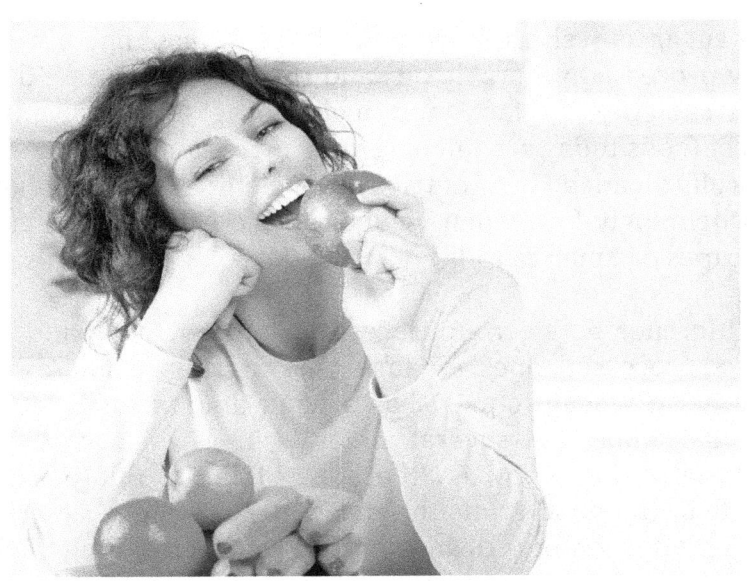

Chapter 2

Getting Nude for Beauty

If you are going to be as beautiful as possible- both inside and out- then your diet should be as beautiful as possible too. And the most beautiful of all ways to eat is to get Nude!

Nude is short for "nutrient-dense" and refers to eating foods that are the most concentrated, nutritious sources of specific nutrients. In essence, nutrient-dense foods are the opposite of "empty calories". "Empty" calories are calories (a measure of energy, expressed as units of heat) that are empty of- not accompanied by- nutrients. Classic examples of foods that contain only empty calories are refined white flour and refined white sugar as well as most refined "hard" alcoholic beverages. Highly processed vegetable oils and shortenings also tend to fall in this category. In fact, most highly processed "convenience" and fast foods today are full of refined ingredients that tend to be calorically loaded but nutrient deficient. This is what we overwhelmingly find when we look at the culinary and grocery landscapes of America today.

The difference between unprocessed, "whole" foods and highly refined, processed ones is stark- and startling. For example, whole grain wheat actually has a good amount of B vitamins, vitamin E, fiber, and several minerals in it-which is why it is sometimes referred to as "the staff of life". But when it is processed, the good stuff- the nutrients- are mostly discarded. What is left is empty- dead- flour. It has a nice, long shelf life (even the rodents and cockroaches don't want it!) but has virtually no nutrient value. The same goes for sugar. Whole or raw sugar in its natural state is well supplied with minerals and vitamins, but refined white sugar only has empty calories left-virtually no nutrients survive the process of refinement.

Eating nutrient-dense, or "Nude", is the best way to ensure that you get an abundance of nutrients. By contrast, the standard American diet, or S.A.D. for short, is a highly processed affair and is loaded with preservatives, artificial colors and flavors, synthetic hormones, and other additives. It is also loaded with empty calories. Often some synthetic vitamins are added back in an attempt to restore some of what was lost in a farcical process called "enriching".

The distinction between these two styles of eating is huge. A nutrient-dense diet is far less processed, and emphasizes foods that are typically eaten closer to their natural state. It contains lots of fresh, often raw produce, and is full of natural pigments and colors and intact nutrients including live enzymes.

A nutrient-dense approach to eating also incorporates plenty of "super foods"- foods that are uniquely rich in specific nutrients. A few examples might include almonds with their healthy fiber, protein, and vitamin E, blueberries- rich in antioxidants, fresh flax seed oil- with its abundant levels of alpha-linolenic acid (a vegetarian omega 3 fatty acid), organic salad greens, fresh carrot juice, coconut butter, organic, fresh eggs, raw goat cheese, brown rice, sea weeds such as dulse or kelp, "super-greens" such as spirulina or chlorella, and if you are not vegetarian, foods such as wild salmon, and organic meats like buffalo, lamb, or elk. I also include treats such as dark chocolate and even some microbrew beers as nutrient-dense foods.

My book on weight loss, diet, and metabolism, *The Nutrient-Dense Diet* (www.organichealthyliving.com) contains lots of helpful information about nutrient-dense eating, including recipes and tips on how to transition successfully to a more nutrient-dense way of eating. Eating "Nude" is not a fad or quick-fix diet plan. Rather, it is a sensible, tried and true, ancient way of eating that reflects our need for the highest quality foods possible. And in today's stressful and often toxic world, we need to eat Nude more than ever!

Nutrient-dense eating is easy, empowering, intuitive, and fun. Instead of feeling deprived, eating this way actually celebrates "the goodness of good food". Being open-minded to new foods and seeking them out helps us create a new, far healthier relationship with food; instead of being afraid of food, we can embrace the adventure of eating with joy and pleasure. This is a far more beautiful- and healthy- way to approach food than the adversarial relationship many of us currently have with the S.A.D diet.

What does getting "Nude" look like? It might mean shopping at farmer's markets for fresh grown, local produce, purchasing heirloom and other "exotic" or traditional foods, trading with your neighbor for her tomatoes or her kale or fresh peas. You might spend more of your time shopping in this way, and less time eating pre-cooked, microwavable quick meals or eating "grab and go" snacks at the convenience store or drive through fast food joint.

Eating Nude means we can give up being fat-phobic, carb-phobic, etc. because Nude eating is above all, about *quality*. Let's take fats as an example. Instead of viewing all fats (for example) as "bad", the Nude style of eating focuses on finding the "best", most nutrient-dense fats and oils. In this way, we can eat fats and oils that are actually good for us- nourishing our skin, organs, and our cells' membranes as nature intended. Avocados, fresh grass-fed raw cream butter, coconut oil, flax oil, or hemp oil are examples of healthy, good-for-us fats and oils. Similarly, we can find good carbs- and enjoy them as well without so much guilt or worry. Nude eating restores our confidence in good food, and allows us to relax around food. No more worry lines!

This is how it should be. In recent decades we have become embroiled in a sort of war with food. We debate about it, worry about it, stress about it, and obsess about it. But our food needn't be our "enemy". Instead we need to re-create a healthier, more intelligent approach to our food choices. Food should be here to nourish, aid, help, and support us in our lives. Simply understanding the fundamental- and pretty obvious- differences between what is natural, safe, and good for our bodies and what is unnatural, manipulated, and highly questionable should provide us with a common sense approach to that most ancient of human impulses- how to nourish ourselves.

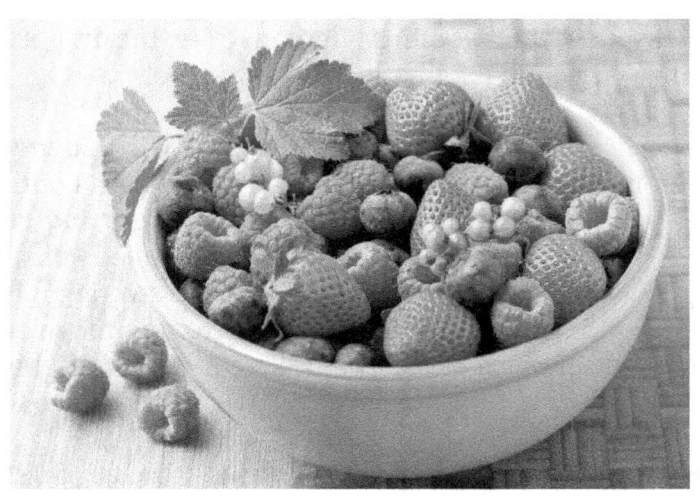

Chapter 3

Specific Nude Foods for Beauty

Getting Nude for beauty is easy! Because the emphasis in eating this way is always about quality, the Nude eating plan is actually more pleasurable and satisfying than eating in a "fast food", conventional way. While for some there is a definite adjustment- we all can get quite attached to our habits- even bad ones- many find that having permission to "get Nude" is a great relief and joy. The nutrient-dense diet actually opens one up to a whole new world of wonderful culinary opportunities.

Much of the Nude diet is about freshness. Raw, live foods with all their vibrancy and color left intact makes up a large portion of the Nude diet. Colorful, flavorful, and fresh produce such as in-season fruits and crisp flavorful veggies are given a large center stage in the Nude diet. Beautiful salads- brimming with a variety of veggies and other goodies- demonstrate the importance of adding diversity and imagination to a great diet.

The basic idea behind getting Nude for beauty is that we need to be as well-nourished and well supplied with healthy nutrients as possible in order to keep making the healthiest and strongest tissues to replace worn out, diseased, or stressed cells, tissues, and organs. We also need to keep ourselves strong and healthy in order to be able to best cope with any environmental stressors and influences that could have a detrimental effect on our bodies.

As I mentioned, raw, fresh produce is one of the cornerstones to the Nude eating plan for being beautiful from within. Fresh fruit and fresh salads are both undeniably important and should be enjoyed as much as possible. My preference is definitely to purchase organically grown produce when possible and affordable, but if only conventional produce is available, that is certainly acceptable!

Another important and highly enjoyable way to enjoy fresh produce is to juice it! Getting a juicer and making fresh fruit juice, fresh veggie juice such as carrot juice, or a blend is a superb way of getting concentrated amounts of nutrients into your body. Along with the minerals and vitamins in fresh juice, you will also be ingesting an abundance of *enzymes*- small but important protein-like molecules that are only associated with live or living foods. Since "we are what we eat" I always say that eating live (aka "raw") foods is the best way to "wake up" your cells. If your food is fresh and alive, then your health, your body, your cells, and your life will be alive and vibrant as well. You don't have to become a raw "foodist" or fanatic in order to be Nude, but I definitely would encourage you to check out and share in their enthusiasm. Incorporating plenty of raw foods in your diet can definitely increase the glow from within that comes from you radiating great health!

I am also a big fan of the "right" fats. Many Americans have become what I call "fat phobic"- associating all kinds of health problems with fat. But the truth is, not all fats are bad for you and in reality, we actually require the good ones to be optimally healthy. In fact, most bad fats are those associated with the S.A.D diet. Fried, overheated fats, margarines and trans fats, and over-processed, refined oils are not good for you at all, and may in fact be quite detrimental. On the other hand, really fresh, good oils can do amazing things for your body, immune system, and vitality.

Our cells *all* require healthy lipids (fats and oils). Cell membranes in particular and other cellular structures need high quality fats. In particular your mitochondria- the special "energy factories" within each cell that literally burn calories in order to produce our cellular energy - require the proper fats in order to operate at peak efficiency. The nervous system and our immune systems also need the right oils and fats in adequate amounts. In addition, many hormones and other important bio- molecules are made in part or wholly out of essential lipids. The truth is, however, that most American diets are quite deficient in high quality, essential oils while being overloaded with the bad ones.

A proper nutrient-dense diet can supply these healthy oils with ease. Some of the many sources of high quality lipids include many cold water fish oils, flax seed oil, avocados, organic butter, virgin olive oil, and many raw (not roasted) nuts and seeds, such as almonds, walnuts, hemp seeds, pumpkin seeds, and sunflower seeds. Coconut oil is also a wonderful food that is completely safe and beneficial. Some of these oils can be taken as a supplement, but others are easily- and deliciously- incorporated into nutrient-dense meals in the forms of salad dressings and in many other creative ways.

Trace minerals are also important components in the Nude eating plan. Many people love to incorporate dulse, nori, kelp, and other seaweeds (sometimes affectionately called "sea vegetables") since they are such great sources of trace minerals from the oceans. Such minerals add to the elemental diversity within our bodies and may provide further resilience to disease and stress. As we shall see, some of these are crucial for the proper development and optimal health of our "beauty tissues"- our hair, skin, and nails.

Finally, quality proteins are a must in the *Beautiful from Within* program. Hair, skin, and nails are all made largely from proteins- and proteins are assembled within the body from circulating amino acids, which ultimately come from our dietary proteins. While all protein sources supply us with amino acids to re-use, many researchers feel that the added hormones, antibiotics, and other agricultural chemicals in conventionally raised beef, poultry, pork, and dairy render these less than desirable protein sources. For this important reason, I strongly recommend only eating meat, eggs, and dairy from organically raised and humanely treated animals *if* you are going to eat meat and animal products.

In addition to the general recommendations listed above, there are also several highly touted "beauty" foods that may have especially useful properties. Blueberries and pomegranates are two very popular fruits that contain high levels of important anti-oxidants. As we will discuss later, anti-oxidants help to protect sensitive tissues from the destructive effects of oxygen, chemicals, and UV light. Many of the more colorful fruits (purple, red, and bluish berries especially) and vegetables are renowned for having high levels of these beneficial substances.

Tomatoes and tomato sauces are also considered to be very protective due to the presence of yet another important pigment- the red colored lycopene. Lycopene may have protective properties for the skin in particular, and may prevent skin damage and premature aging due to burns and UV exposure. In addition to tomatoes, good dietary sources of lycopene include watermelon and guava fruit.

I could have mentioned eggs in the protein section, but these nutritional wonders have so much to offer as a beauty food that they really stand alone as a uniquely special Nude food. Eggs offer much more than just protein-though the protein in eggs is considered to be of the highest quality. Eggs are also one of the best sources of "biological sulfur". Sulfur is an important and crucial component of some of the most important skin, hair, and nail proteins: keratin. You will read more about sulfur in a later chapter.

Of course everyone knows eggs are a contributor of cholesterol as well- but fewer know that cholesterol is actually a very desirable and beneficial nutrient- one that our bodies wisely utilize in several important ways. For decades the medical profession has done a good job at making us fearful of cholesterol, but now we know that cholesterol actually does much good and deserves our respect and appreciation.

Cholesterol is a special molecule- and its unique shape and properties have made it a vital "precursor" molecule. This simply means that cholesterol acts as a key starting point for the manufacture of other biologically important molecules. In reality cholesterol is actually an essential "building block" for the biosynthesis of several super important hormones. All of the sex hormones- which means, testosterone, the estrogens, and natural progesterone- are synthesized directly from cholesterol in our bodies. Similarly, cholesterol is the beginning molecule in a series of biochemical reactions that leads ultimately to the production of vitamin D-which allows the absorption of calcium to take place. The stress and anti-inflammatory corticosteroids, such as cortisone, are also synthesized from cholesterol molecule building blocks. So, far from being something to be afraid of, cholesterol is in reality essential for our health and for life itself.

A few quick cautionary words about eggs though. First, the conventional commercial poultry industry is renowned for employing very large quantities of veterinary pharmaceutical drugs, including a wide variety of antibiotics and estrogenic hormones among others. My strong advice is to *only* purchase eggs from truly free-range, properly raised and fed hens. I feel there is *a huge* difference in the end product in terms of the presence or virtual absence of these chemicals in conventional versus organic eggs.

My second piece of advice concerns *how* your eggs are prepared. Very high temperatures may oxidize or damage sensitive cholesterol molecules and other nutrients in eggs, rendering them less beneficial or even hazardous. As boiling is a much lower temperature cooking method compared to frying, I advise that most of your egg consumption be from eggs that have been boiled- whether hard boiled, soft boiled, or poached.

And please remember, factory-farmed, mass-produced hens- and their eggs- are raised under quite horrific conditions. I really believe that we ingest a lot of things along with our food. Cruelty and suffering should not be one of them! Free-range eggs are best. Being informed as to the reality of how some of our food is raised is an important part of being wise, responsible participants in how we nourish ourselves!

Another vitally important nutrient for the skin is vitamin C. Vitamin C acts as an important anti-oxidant, but its importance as a beauty nutrient goes well beyond that role. The deeper value of Vitamin C is due to its role in collagen synthesis. Collagen is a critical connective tissue, and gives elasticity, firmness, and contours to many areas of the body. Vitamin C-containing foods including citrus and many other fruits are therefore extremely powerful beauty-from-within foods. These fruits and vegetables also contribute other significant nutrients, including minerals, some vitamins, and in particular enzymes and colorful pigments that themselves typically act as anti-oxidants- free radical scavengers that may help slow down tissue inflammation and damage and therefore the aging process itself. Eating lots of fresh, juicy, colorful fruits and vegetables is a very healthy, Nude-and enjoyable- way to eat and nourish ourselves.

One of the most enjoyable aspects of getting Nude for beauty is the sheer amount of wonderful, nutritious, delicious food available. One thing that is commonly heard from people who are new to eating healthily is their concern that there will be "nothing good to eat". Fear of the unknown is perfectly normal, and the idea of leaving behind the comforts and familiarity of a lifetime of eating and shopping habits can naturally lead to doubts, insecurity, hesitancy, and concerns. The good news though, is that becoming a Nude-ist (eater) can be a gradual process and journey and therefore doesn't have to be a total shock. In *The Nutrient-Dense Diet* I discuss some of the ways that nutrient-dense foods can be introduced into one's diet gradually, therefore slowly but surely increasing the nutritional quality of one's diet bit by bit.

Best Beauty Foods

- Almonds, most nuts, seeds (nut butters like almond butter)
- Avocados
- Bee pollen
- Coconut oil
- Dark Chocolate
- Eggs/organic! (poached, hard boiled, soft boiled)
- Flax oil
- Fresh Fruits (berries, pomegranates, mangos, kiwi, etc)
- Fresh Juices (carrot, beet, celery, ginger, lemon, apple)
- Kombucha
- Nutritional yeast
- Leafy greens
- Legumes and lentils
- Matcha Green Tea
- Nutritional yeast
- Olives, oil
- Sea vegetables (sea weeds)
- Sardines
- Sauerkraut (raw)
- Spices/herbs
- Spirulina
- Turmeric
- Veggies (all; raw, steamed, lightly stir fried)
- Whole grains (brown rice, quinoa, millet, oats)
- Wild salmon

Super Fruits for Super Health

Since we truly are what we eat, for the most vibrant beauty and health we should eat plenty of fresh, colorful, live fruits. Fresh fruit gives us needed vitamins, minerals, enzymes (living proteins found only in uncooked or "raw" live foods), fiber, and other nutrients such as anti-oxidant molecules. Additionally fresh fruit also supplies us with color (pigments), flavor, fun, and sweetness that can help us resist eating less healthy processed sugars. And, almost everyone knows that all fruits are great sources of vitamin C- the important "beauty vitamin" that plays an important role in collagen synthesis to help us look young and stay firm.

Cherries

We all need adequate refreshing sleep to look and feel our best and cherries just might be a delicious way to get a great night's sleep! New research has shown that tart cherry juice helps improve both the quality and quantity of sleep as well as reducing insomnia symptoms in some people. Cherries are also potent anti-inflammatory aids and may benefit athletes and others with symptoms of joint pain, mild arthritis, etc. Whether fresh, dried, or as juice, cherries can be a delicious way to keep on top of things in your quest for health and quality of life.

Pomegranates

Research on pomegranates continues to shed light on the amazing array of health benefits associated with this queen of fruits. Among many other benefits, unique molecules found in pomegranates called punicalagins effectively suppress harmful collagen-attacking inflammatory enzymes. Collagen is one of the body's most important "beauty proteins" so protecting it from harm's way is a key strategy in promoting true "beauty from within".

Cranberries

Cranberries have been extensively studied for many years and our understanding of the numerous benefits of these tart little berries continues to expand. Women have known for years that cranberries have documented benefits in counteracting urinary tract infections. One of the ways they accomplish this is through a unique compound that reduces the ability of the bad bacteria to cling to the walls of the urinary tract so they cannot form colonies and grow. The benefits of cranberries are numerous: in addition to having anti-adhesive properties, they are also anti microbial, anti-inflammatory, and anti-oxidant. But they are completely pro-health and beauty!

Apples

In this era of exotic new "super fruits" the original health food- the apple- seems to have lost some of its aura of specialness. However, apples are being shown fresh respect, as much research is taking a fresh look at the many benefits apples possess. Apples are high in an important anti-inflammatory compound called quercetin, which is a very beneficial bioflavonoid with a ton of good research behind it. Apples are also famous for their pectin content. Pectin is a soluble fiber, and has long been associated with lowering cholesterol levels.

New research is also shifting focus to the peel- where the vast majority of nutrients reside. Because pesticide residues tend to stay on the outside of the fruit, it is always best to play it safe and purchase organic apples. And don't forget- this is good general advice for all types of fruits as well!

The Beauty of an Open Mind

Getting Nude is actually a fun adventure if you approach it with the right attitude. In one's eating habits, as in most everything in life, having an open mind usually rewards us with new experiences, and enriches us in multitudes of ways. There is a hugely diverse and fascinating world of foods and tastes out there, and trying new and nutritious items expands our world, makes us more interesting people, and generally rewards us by broadening our horizons. And, by enjoying and eating a wider range of foods we potentially expand the opportunities to ingest a wider array of nutrients such as more exotic phytonutrients, plant pigments, and other molecules that might bring positive chemical and energetic messages into our bodies. As we keep being reminded, if "we are what we eat", then eating a more diverse number of foods might make us more diverse and interesting people ourselves. And what could be more beautiful than that?

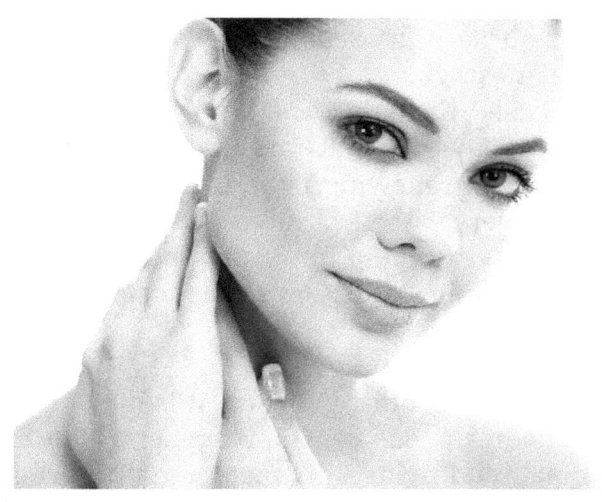

Chapter 4

Your Skin: Touching Your World

Your skin is your body's largest organ. It is also your most visible. It is your boundary with the world, and your biggest and most important sense organ. Our skin protects us, gives us valuable feedback about our world, and senses and distinguishes heat, cold, pressure, pain, and of course, pleasure. Your skin is your single biggest beauty asset, and clearly reflects the nutritional status of your body. As one of the main portals of detoxification and elimination, your skin is often asked to do a lot of work in order to keep you clean and (relatively) unpolluted. Fortunately, your largest and most sensual organ will respond beautifully to the nutritional support and loving kindness you show it.

Although the skin is our largest organ, it is also the thinnest, and in some ways, the most vulnerable. Composed of just a few handfuls of layers of cells, the outermost layer, or epidermis, and the deeper, or dermal layer of cells are specialized protective tissues that are constantly renewing, or rejuvenating themselves. Of course this is a very practical thing, as our bodies are continually bumping and rubbing up against our environment- our car seats, our beds, our clothes- even the water in our tubs or showers.

With so much friction and contact going on, it is no wonder that the surface of our bodies needs constant replacing. Continually growing, wearing out, and dying, this means that the cells that comprise our skin give us an accurate and honest accounting of what we have- and haven't- been doing for them. The great news here is that we can always begin today providing the next generation of cells- next week's or next month's skin- with the raw materials needed for a fresh and beautiful start.

Although it appears deceptively simple, your skin is actually home to a wide variety of cells and tissue types. Though the majority of your skin is comprised of the common, flattened, epithelial type cells, other cell types abound as well. Tiny hair follicles, even tinier muscle cells (which contract to cause you to have goose bumps), sensitive nerve endings (for both pain and pleasure), and miniscule blood vessels- the capillaries- all make up the larger community of tissue types that we collectively refer to as our "skin". In addition the skin contains sweat and oil glands, various amounts of pigment, and all the biochemical switches and factories necessary to manufacture many of the compounds of life. With such diversity and specialization of cell types and an array of functions, it is clearly important that we do not take our precious skin for granted!

Preserving Your Beautiful Skin

A massage therapist friend of mine recently remarked how "challenged" the skin of many of the people she worked on was. She mentioned in particular the prevalence of dry skin, but she also related to me how common it is to see tough, leathery skin, skin with eczema, psoriasis, rashes of all kinds, fungal infections, and other changes in texture and signs of aging. Smooth, soft, silky skin is apparently not as common as we'd like to think. Why?

As we have seen, our skin is where we interface with the external environment. And, as if there aren't enough harsh threats from our environment, there is the added insult of all too often not being adequately nourished from within. Let's take a closer look at this double jeopardy, and see what we can do to protect our skin from without, while nourishing it from within.

We all have heard the constantly repeated warnings to avoid excessive sun exposure. Yet the burning rays of ultraviolet radiation are only one of many insults that your skin is vulnerable to. And surprisingly, it may not be the biggest threat that your skin faces. In fact, for some, too little sun exposure can be a bigger health threat than too much- for the skin (and for our health as a whole) a delicate balance with the sun must exist- too much and we burn; too little, and we deprive our bodies of vitamin D, an essential hormone/vitamin important for the absorption of calcium, bone health, and immune strength as well.

Frying is not an option- virtually all skin experts agree that the damaging rays of the sun can increase your risk for skin cancer as well as generally accelerating the aging ("weathering") of the skin. How does this take place? Ionizing radiation from the sun promotes the generation and activity within the skin's tissues of free radicals – unbalanced molecular forms of oxygen with free electrons which hungrily attack vulnerable cell structures, such as cell membranes. Such damaged cell structures will never look or act as young and healthy as undamaged tissue. But besides the effects of solar radiation, other compounds and substances can attack skin tissue as well. One of the worst is an everyday chemical that is awfully hard to avoid- chlorine.

In today's world, chlorine is every bit as hard to avoid as the sun. In fact it may be even harder to avoid given how much time most of us spend indoors nowadays. Used to sterilize water and other surfaces, chlorine is added to virtually every municipal water supply in the U.S., meaning we- our skin- contacts it every time we bathe, shower, rinse our face, or take a plunge in a pool or hot tub. Chlorine is a very harsh, drying chemical, and is a potent creator of free radicals. Sensitive skin and sensitive parts of your body may therefore react to the chlorine in your home or at the pool or Jacuzzi by becoming excessively dry or even irritated. Chlorine is probably the least suspected common environmental irritant our skin faces in day-to-day life. And it is precisely because it is so common that we typically overlook it and suspect other culprits for our skin problems.

So what to do if you suspect chlorine is a major cause in your skin's challenging life? As I said, chlorine is hard to avoid- but there are solutions. One step that more and more people are taking is installing a chlorine-removing water filter- or several- in their home. Different technologies with differing capabilities are available, and I suggest you find the best possible type for your budget. Why spend countless dollars on creams and lotions if the original problem is coming out of your tap or shower head? Depending upon your needs and budget, you could either purchase a filter for your shower or consider a "whole house" option.

Outside of your home the most important thing is to be as aware as possible- and your nose may be your best guide. Chlorine has a familiar, strong chemical smell, and levels in public water supplies can vary widely. If your nose alerts you to the fact that chlorine has been freshly added to the spa or pool, you might be better off avoiding going in; your caution could reward your skin (and hair and scalp) with extra mileage. This should make sense to us; if we avoid extra ultraviolet light because it is damaging, shouldn't we avoid excess chlorine for the same reason?

Chlorine levels can fluctuate widely- if the treatment plant near your home or club has just added it (some plants add it at specific, regular intervals), levels could be higher before they taper off. And pools, hot tubs, and the like can also vary tremendously. Most European spas don't even use this harsh and toxic chemical; instead they sterilize their water with a combination of safer, less toxic techniques, such as treating their water with hydrogen peroxide and ultra violet light.

The other biggest threats to your skin come from your lifestyle choices. Whatever adds to the load of free radicals in our bodies will definitely be reflected in the quality of your skin. And while free radicals from UV light and chlorine are huge problems, two other contributors to the free radical load in your body are important to consider: smoking and drinking.

Smoking and drinking are two of the biggest risk factors cited by doctors for increasing our chances of contracting certain cancers, including cancers of the epithelial tissues. Everyone has seen the signs of premature aging in people who have been long term heavy smokers or drinkers. The best beauty advice anyone can be given who has one or both of these habits is: quit! If you do drink, please do so moderately; the best form of alcohol from an overall health standpoint is definitely red wine. Red wine at least has some very beneficial antioxidants, including one,

31

resveratrol which is reputed to have certain anti-aging properties. "Hard" liquors, by contrast, such as whiskeys, brandy, bourbon, and the like contain some very potent cancer-causing chemicals, called "urethanes". Urethanes are a byproduct of distilling, and spirits containing higher levels of these molecules may be an under recognized major health risk. Why chance it?

The other lifestyle factor that can negatively affect the appearance of the skin is heavy sugar consumption. Sugar has many deleterious effects within the body, but what nutritionists and other scientists have discovered is that the skin and other tissues can be affected by high blood sugar levels in interesting ways. Molecules of sugar can attach or stick to certain proteins in the skin and other tissues to cause cumbersome problems. Such "sticky proteins" are less efficient at being metabolized properly and can build up as unsightly deposits, such as "liver spots" or aging blemishes in the skin. In fact some scientists even suspect similar sticky proteins (called "plaques") are responsible for some of the neurological problems in the brain associated with aging. Attaching sugar to protein in this way is a chemical reaction or process called "glycation". And the association of this process with aging is easy to remember: scientists call these sticky proteins "advanced glycation end -products" or AGESs! So if you don't want to age prematurely, cut back on the sugar. Your skin for one doesn't really need it!

Along with too many refined carbohydrates, the other food - sourced threat to skin health can come from the wrong type of fats. Fats are actually a complex, broad family of molecules, called lipids, that are characterized by their general insolubility in water. Often (unjustly) maligned, the spectrum of fats in our diets runs the gamut from very healthy and highly desirable to very unhealthy and highly undesirable. Good fats are vital to health and do all sorts of positive things in our bodies, from building healthy cell membranes to being the source molecules and building blocks for certain hormones, neurotransmitters, and many other structures. On the other hand, bad fats contribute toxic free-radicals, and can "gum up the works" by interfering with normal cellular structures and functions. Such bad fats should definitely be avoided if one sincerely wants to get the most out of the *beautiful from within* program.

What are the worst offenders in the bad fats category? In general we can say that any fat that is highly refined, processed, and/or heated has been turned into a bad fat. Basically, this means most deep fried (very highly heated) oils and the foods that are cooked in them. Unfortunately this includes many of our favorite snack foods and treats. Yes, I am referring to potato chips, onion rings, and other greasy, deep fried foods like fried chicken, etc. Most of us love these crispy, greasy foods- I have spent many moments in store aisles, gazing wistfully and longingly at the many seductive bags of chips of all kinds. But in the end, (usually) will power- and common sense- win out, and I walk away, empty handed, but happy knowing I am doing my body a big favor by not succumbing to the crunchy, crispy, greasy treats.

The other major types of bad fats are the heavily processed oils that become transformed into hydrogenated oils. Most of us know by now that hydrogenated fats are chemically altered oils that have had their molecular structure altered to change their melting point (making them spreadable solids at room temperature instead of liquid). This chemical process is a pretty harsh treatment and many of the resultant (partially) hydrogenated fats are changed from what scientists call their natural "cis" configuration to the unnatural "trans" form. This is why so many products now are being reformulated by the food industry to be "trans-fat free". However, it still pays to read labels; while much of the food industry is taking measures to remove partially hydrogenated oils and trans-fats from their recipes, many products still contain them. Lipid-rich skin tissues will uptake whatever fatty acids are available from the fats circulating in the blood stream. This is a clear example of the statement, "you are what you eat". If you eat food that contains hydrogenated oils, they will be absorbed into your bloodstream and ultimately end up in different cells in your body, including your skin. Unhealthy fats make unhealthy cells, tissues, and skin. Pretty simple!

Nutrition and Your Skin

Vitamin C

One of the best friends your skin has is easy to get and easier to enjoy. It is good, old fashioned vitamin C! As we have seen earlier, vitamin C, or ascorbic acid, is the most important water-soluble antioxidant in the body. This means vitamin C helps in the all-important job of neutralizing the harmful free-radicals that seek to damage membranes and other structures in our body's tissues, such as the skin.

But vitamin C has another, equally impressive role to play in the health of your body and in particular in the health of your skin: it is the source of that all-important beauty molecule, collagen.

Collagen is a specialized protein that is also considered a type of "connective tissue". As a connective tissue, collagen helps to hold other tissues together, and gives shape and contour to our bodies. Collagen also helps to hold structures firmly in place, so they don't sag or become loose. That is why scurvy or severe vitamin C deficiency can result in the loosening of our teeth in their sockets- because the connective tissue that is supposed to hold the teeth firmly in place weakens or vanishes.

In the same way, a lack of adequate vitamin C also weakens the strength of our capillaries, leading to an increased tendency for them to bruise or bleed easily. Varicose veins and hemorrhoids are both due to weak veins so vitamin C might help in some of these situations too. So in addition to giving us full lips, collagen helps make our bodies stronger, more elastic, and more resilient in a wide variety of ways.

Interestingly, both smoking and excessive drinking deplete our bodies of vitamin C, further reasons to avoid or reduce these habits. Ascorbic acid is also diminished by exposure to other harsh chemicals- in an attempt to neutralize or detoxify free radicals our vitamin C is used up, leaving little or none for our body's reserves.

Of course, vitamin C is widely available in supplement form, but it is even better to get it as nature intended- through our food. Ascorbic acid is abundant in fruits and many vegetables, but is pretty much totally absent from processed and over-cooked foods. Coffee, sodas, and sweets have virtually no ascorbic acid, so the best beauty advice one can receive, nutritionally, is to eat plenty of fresh fruit and other produce. In fact, not smoking, avoiding as many harsh chemicals as possible, drinking several glasses a day of pure water, and eating at least several servings of fresh fruit daily is a great core approach to staying as young looking and healthy as possible!

Although vitamin C is crucial for the *Beautiful from Within* program, fresh produce has numerous other virtues in addition to its ascorbic acid. In a strong supportive role, numerous other molecules in produce also act as potent anti-oxidants, synergizing with vitamin C. In particular bioflavonoids, molecules called phenols, and the bright pigments in fresh produce all have an important function in helping keep harmful free-radicals from doing their damage.

Sulfur and Zinc:

Sulfur and zinc are both very important minerals involved in skin health and vibrancy. In fact, I consider both to be highly significant "beauty minerals". Both are involved in skin health, but the same is true for their roles in hair and nail health as well.

The vast majority of proteins are characterized by the presence of the element nitrogen in their amino acid make-up so protein supplies us with the nitrogen atoms for our bodies' proteins that in general, fats and carbohydrates don't typically contain. But in addition to nitrogen, a few amino acids are reliant on another element that is not found in too many other classes of molecules. And that element is sulfur.

As it turns out, hair, skin, and nails are all composed of molecular compounds that utilize sulfur. The protein keratin, for example, which makes up virtually all of your hair's protein, is rich in sulfur-containing amino acids, which is the exact reason why burning hair smells like cooked eggs or a struck match- each contains a lot of biologically active sulfur in their chemical make-up.

Sulfur is found in a number of foods: the cabbage family, which also includes broccoli, Brussels sprouts and cauliflower among other plant foods is a good source of biologically available sulfur. So too is the allium family. Allium foods that can contribute sulfur to the "beauty cause" include garlic, onions, shallots, and leeks. Finally, eggs are an excellent source of biological sulfur as much of egg white protein (albumin) contains a large percentage of important sulfur-containing amino acids.

Zinc is also an extremely important mineral nutrient that is required throughout the body for a wide range of functions. One of the most important of its many functions is its essential role in protein synthesis. Without adequate zinc, protein molecules cannot be assembled properly. Since your skin (as well as your hair and nails) are all largely composed of proteins, zinc is crucial for resupplying and replacing worn out tissues. Zinc is also critical for successful wound healing. Zinc is present in a wide range of foods, but many of the best sources, such as oysters and pumpkin seeds are not frequently consumed by many people. Therefore, zinc supplements are something to strongly consider in your *beautiful from within* program. A good average daily dose for many adults is in the 25mg-50mg range.

Silica:

Many researchers are starting to take notice of silica's roles in human health. Silica is actually the most common mineral in the earth's crust, and is a major component in sand and quartz. Like carbon and oxygen, life on earth has always co-existed with silica and silicate compounds. In many plants, silicate molecules are responsible for increasing the structural strength of the plant's stems and other structures, and evidence is steadily increasing that silica molecules play a similar part in the structural integrity and strength of hair, skin, and nail tissue in humans as well. Silica comes from plant sources, so people who don't eat much produce may have sub-optimal levels as they age. And we should keep in mind that many soils that our food is grown on these days may be depleted of certain minerals, including silica. In addition, hydroponically or greenhouse grown foods my contain little or none of this mineral.

Silica levels are definitely known to decline in the body as we age, and since absorption of silica is generally not that great, many people advocate supplementation as a way to ensure that enough biologically available silica is ingested. In youth, higher silica levels are associated with strong connective tissue, blood vessel wall integrity, and bone strength.

As far as skin goes, silica is known to complex (or join) with important molecules known as glycosaminoglycans, which are closely linked to collagen and connective tissue formation. Aging skin might be helped- especially its elasticity, thickness, and strength- through silica supplementation. Wound healing is another possible area that silica supplementation may help. In Europe and other parts of the world, many women take precautionary silica supplements to help ensure youthful, healthy, and strong skin. As a bonus, silica is also strongly linked to the other important beauty tissues: strong hair and nails. Depending upon the soil in which they are grown, many plants can be rich sources of silica. One of the most famous is the herb known as horsetail, which has been used for centuries as a hair and skin tonic.

Selenium and Vitamin E:

Like vitamin C, the mineral selenium is an important antioxidant that is thought to offer protection against cell damage caused by free radicals. Some excellent research has shown that selenium, along with vitamin E, might help reduce the risk of some skin cancers. The most nutrient-dense dietary source of selenium is brazil nuts, but whole grains, seafood, and eggs are also good sources. Natural vitamin E is found in spinach, avocados, almonds, sunflower seeds, and wheat germ oil.

Essential Fatty Acids:

Next on our list of the most important skin nutrients are the essential fatty acids (or EFAs). Such vitally important oils are ideally sourced as fresh and natural and possible, and are best taken internally as unheated, minimally processed (unrefined) oils. These nutrients are extremely crucial for *BFW* skin. The omega 3 fatty acids in particular are famous for their anti-inflammatory properties as well as their role in immune health. Such oils are quite fragile and perishable. I recommend buying only truly cold-pressed oils that are stored in refrigeration and sold in amber glass bottles or a high quality inert opaque plastic.

Well-nourished, healthy cells have to have healthy membranes- those lipid-rich boundaries that are essentially the "skin" of each cell. Fish oils from cod and some other species are the richest sources of the essential omega 3 fatty acids. For vegetarians, cold pressed flax seed oil or a good blend of flax with some additional oils is a great way to go for superbly well-nourished skin cells. In addition to flax seeds, hemp seeds, chia seeds, and black walnuts are also excellent sources of vegetarian source omega 3 fats. Avocados also provide good quality, "live" oils.

Omega 3 fats may also help the skin retain moisture and can contribute to a softer, less dry appearance by the skin. Dry, and inflamed skin may also benefit dramatically from increasing your intake of these beneficial oils. In some cases, skin disorders such as eczema and psoriasis have been known to improve from taking such oils. The typical American diet (S.A.D) is known to be extremely deficient in these important nutrients.

Vitamin A and the Carotenoids

Vitamin A is also an extremely important nutrient for skin health. Vitamin A deficiencies are well known to manifest as dry, flaky, or scaly skin. Though vitamin A is plentiful in many animal foods including butter, whole milk, cream, and egg yolks, it is thought that many people still don't get adequate or optimal amounts- and of course vegans and some vegetarians may be at an even greater risk.

Beta carotene is a precursor of Vitamin A, and is abundant in many orange and yellow vegetables such as squashes and carrots- however some people simply aren't as efficient in converting it to the actual vitamin form of the molecule. As a result, many nutritionists and physicians recommend taking a vitamin A supplement to ensure optimal levels.

Beta carotene is probably the best known of the molecular family known as the carotenoids- yellow and orange pigmented compounds that are found in a wide variety of vegetables and other foods. Part of an anti-aging "beautiful from within" skin care program should definitely keep these molecules in mind. Carrot juice is an excellent way to get a good concentrated dose.

Solar radiation, coupled with certain environmental provocateurs, can cause oxidative and genetic changes that can lead to photo-aging and even skin cancers such as melanoma. Premature or exaggerated wrinkles, sagging, dryness, discoloration, and age spots may all result from a lifetime of (over) exposure to the sun and elements. Living near or at the ocean and spending a lot of time on the water or at the beach with the combination of sun, wind, and drying salt can be especially hard on the skin.

As we have discussed, dietary anti-oxidants (i.e. ascorbic acid, tocopherols, alpha lipoic acid, polyphenols from fruits, etc.) are a promising therapeutic and preventive approach to counteract photo-aging in humans. The carotenoids from food are especially known to be deposited in the skin, where they may offer protection against excessive sun exposure. One study, from the National Cancer Institute showed that subjects with higher intakes for Vitamin D, lutein (a phytonutrient found in some vegetables) and total carotenoids had a "significantly reduced risk for melanoma" onset. In animal studies, increasing lutein and zeaxanthin (another carotenoid) helped delay and limit sunburn damage- an exciting find! Yet another carotenoid, lycopene, a reddish pigment found in tomatoes, guava and watermelon, has had similar beneficial and protective effects on the skin. Other positive benefits from lutein and zeaxanthin included enhancing skin elasticity and skin hydration in addition to sunburn protection.

B complex:

Though perhaps not specific to the skin, it is undeniable that the B vitamins are crucial for total body health. Virtually every cell, tissue, and organ in the body relies on adequate levels of all of the B vitamins in order to stay healthy. Many of the B vitamins are involved in the production of energy from carbohydrates, fats, and proteins, and in their absence, cells and tissues may suffer from an energy deficit. Rapidly dividing cells (like the skin's epithelial cells) that must continually grow and reproduce to replace worn out or damaged cells need B vitamins such as folic acid and others in order to reproduce properly and efficiently.

Copper:

Copper is one of the most important minerals in the body- and is responsible for (among many other things) much of our outward appearance as well as our safety within. Copper is intimately involved in bodily processes as diverse as the formation of hemoglobin within red blood cells and the strength and resilience of the aortic wall and the other major blood vessels. But for *BFW* readers, copper's powerful influence over the skin's performance is what is really interesting.

Copper binds with small protein fragments called peptides to create unique copper-peptide complexes that can have an interesting influence over how wounds heal. As it turns out, these complexes actually also have a very positive effect on scar formation- they reduce scarring! The way they do this is still being studied, but it appears that copper peptides can affect collagen deposition in positive ways. They also seem to have anti-inflammatory and anti/dermal irritation properties too, which may indicate that they can slow skin aging through neutralizing free radicals. And another study demonstrated copper peptides stimulated new collagen synthesis better than Retin A.

Another important beauty aspect of copper is that it is a part of the melanin molecule. Melanin is the pigment that gives color and richness to not only our skin, but our hair and even our eyes!

It turns out that copper is truly an underappreciated trace mineral- yet it has so many key functions in our bodies that it truly qualifies as one of the most important of all the health and beauty nutrients. Let's review its roles:

- Copper is directly involved in collagen formation. Collagen is a structural protein, and is important for the integrity of skin, bone, cartilage, tendons, and ligaments.

- Copper helps the body utilize other essential minerals, including iron and zinc

- Copper works intimately with several key antioxidant enzymes- helping to diminish the harmful effects of certain destructive free radicals

- Copper has powerful and important anti-inflammatory properties and is useful in mitigating the effects of some arthritis.

- Copper is necessary for hemoglobin formation and can help in some cases of anemia

- Copper is important and vital for a healthy immune system

- Copper is essential for melanin production

- Copper is necessary in the proper amounts to help prevent osteoporosis

So where do we obtain copper from in our diets? Copper is available in a wide array of foods, although usually in very small amounts. Therefore a varied, nutrient-dense diet will be helpful in ensuring an adequate intake of this important beauty mineral. Some of the many nutrient-dense sources of copper include organ meats, seafood, wheat germ, walnuts and other seeds and nuts (cashews and brazil nuts are good sources), and legumes. Whole grains also supply small amounts. For many people a copper supplement might be a good idea, especially if you are already taking zinc as a supplement. This is because too much zinc can upset the balance of copper in the body and potentially create a deficiency.

If copper is so important to our looks and our health, what are some potential warning signs of an impending deficiency state? Some health symptoms of copper deficiency can include (some cases of) anemia, low body temperature, osteoporosis, increased vulnerability to infections, elevated cholesterol levels, and some cases of thyroid disorders. Beauty issues that may be linked to suboptimal copper intakes can include dry skin, hair problems including brittle hair and hair loss, and premature loss of hair color as well as loss of pigment (color or tone) from the skin. It is also important to mention that long term usage of oral contraceptives has been known to upset copper balances in the body.

Earlier we touched on the important role of unique combinations that copper makes by joining with small protein molecules, called peptides. These copper-peptide "complexes" are reputed by some scientists to renew the skin through a variety of means. According to biochemist Loren Pickart, a researcher who has studied these molecules for many years, copper peptides actually work to smooth wrinkles and age lines by thickening the skin through improving collagen levels as well as by boosting elastin, another important form of connective tissue. Together these molecules may also improve skin moisturization through a combination of strengthening the skin's barrier properties along with raising levels of naturally occurring sugars and proteins (proteoglycans) which, among other things, hold water within the skin's tissue matrix.
If that wasn't enough, there is also evidence that copper peptides can improve the strength and hardness of fingernails through their ability to increase keratinocyte levels. Finally, since copper

peptides are known to have strong anti-inflammatory properties, these molecules may help skin inflammation associated with some forms of acne, rashes, eczema, and rosacea.

In addition to the obvious beauty benefits of copper, this mineral is also of vital importance to our health and longevity as well. It has been long known that copper deficiencies can be associated with early death from hemorrhaging and bursting aneurysms. Since copper is important for keeping blood vessels strong and elastic, many heart disease and cardiovascular disease patients may be suffering from undiagnosed copper deficiencies, and the reasons are related to the same beauty benefits copper can confer, namely its crucial role in improving collagen and elastin levels.

The flexibility and the tensile strength of blood vessels such as arteries, veins, and capillaries are related directly to the quality and quantity of the connective tissue in their walls. Connective tissue provides strength and elasticity and its flexible characteristics allow our blood vessels to "flex" or give with the surges of blood flow. Inflexible, rigid blood vessels are associated with hardening of the arteries, or atherosclerosis (sclerosis literally means, "to harden"). The ability of blood vessels to flex, or "give and take" with surges of blood is directly related to what is measured as "blood pressure". Thus, as we age and our arteries harden and become less flexible, blood pressure can rise, sometimes to dangerous levels. If our vessel walls become weakened, due to poor quality connective tissue in them, then the combination of weak walls and increased pressure can lead to what is known as an aneurysm- a side wall "blow out" much like can happen to an overinflated, worn out tire. Often this is exactly what causes a heart attack (when the blow out occurs within the heart) or a stroke (when the blood vessel that ruptures is in the brain). In legs, weakened vessels may lead to what are commonly known as "varicose" veins; if one occurs in the rectal area; this is what is commonly referred to as "hemorrhoids". All of these conditions have similar causes- weakened vessel walls, often from some combination of factors leading to a rupture or hemorrhage, and often combined with elevated blood pressure.

Nutritional factors clearly offer an important role in each of these situations- not only is copper of vital importance, but as we've seen, vitamin C (ascorbic acid) as well as bioflavonoids can also be of great benefit in strengthening the integrity of vital structures. All contribute in different but synergistic ways to the integrity and strength of blood vessels and other tissues. And through increasing the quality and quantity of collagen and elastin throughout the body, these nutrients contribute directly to our appearance as well as our health and wellness.

Your skin is your largest- and most visible- organ. It reveals to the world a lot about our inner state of health and wellness. Our skin is probably our single biggest "beauty tissue" and the good news is that armed with the right nutritional information, you can take excellent care of your beautiful boundary with the world.

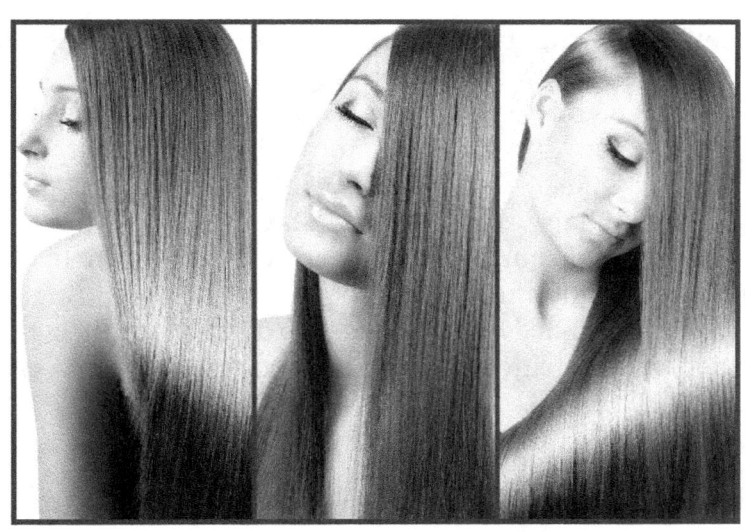

Chapter 5

Healthy, Happy Hair

Hair- that strange beautiful tissue that adorns us, crowns us, and sets us apart- is often the first thing that others notice about us. Our hair is for many our personal fashion statement, and is an immediate clue to others about our sense of style, flair, and even our inner state of health.

Radiant, luxurious, healthy hair can say a lot about our inner health, for it is often a telling reflection of our overall health and wellness. A healthy head of hair attracts potential mates, gives us confidence, and helps us define and set ourselves apart from the crowd. Whether we choose to wear it long, short, or medium; leave it to its natural level of straightness, waviness, or curliness; or whether we straighten it, color it, or curl it- hair is our uniquely human quality- it is the beautiful human version of our feathers, our scales, our wings or our foliage.

Hair can also be one of the most problematic of our tissues. It is all too often too dry, too thin, too brittle, too slow growing, too....troublesome for many of us. Yet like all of our precious body tissues, hair will respond favorably to the proper nourishment and support. While we tend to spend billions of dollars on conditioners, shampoos, perms, coloring, scalp treatments, expensive brushes, etc., most of us give little thought to the very real nutritional needs and requirements that growing hair has.

Hair is the fastest growing tissue in the human body, averaging more than one centimeter per month- and in some individuals, much faster than that. Not surprisingly, like many rapidly dividing cells, hair growth tends to be most robust in young people- peaking for most from age 15-30 or so. In most people hair growth slows down (but doesn't stop) in those 40-50. But hair continues to grow and serve us throughout our lives, and we need to take care of it and honor it throughout our lives if we want to look and feel our best.

Hair is composed almost exclusively of protein, and we will see shortly that this is an important clue in understanding some of the ways to nourish and work with our hair for optimal health. It is also important to understand that hair growth starts from under the scalp skin, in the specialized structures known as hair follicles. Here, tiny blood vessels supply the source nutrients for the growing hair, which needs a constant supply of proteins, essential fatty acids, oxygen, vitamins, and minerals. If the quality of nutrition and blood supply is optimal, and the hormones and other key factors of cell growth are present, then our growing hair can fulfill its promise of healthy, beautiful, and luxurious growth.

Throughout the body, healthy tissue growth depends upon a healthy blood supply- since it is the blood that carries oxygen, and delivers other nutrients to where they are needed. The blood is also crucial for carrying away waste products that can clog or interfere with proper cellular and tissue health. Therefore, the health of our circulatory system is a vital key to the health of our body as a whole. In this way, things that degrade the healthy functioning of our blood vessels- such as smoking, bad fats such as fried oils and hydrogenated (trans fats), too much sugar, etc., also can be detrimental to the health of the hair on our heads.

Similarly, nutrients that are now known to be supportive for arterial health, such as anti-oxidants, good oils (omega 3s), some herbal substances, a fiber and plant rich diet, and certain vitamins and minerals are equally understood to be supportive of healthy hair (and other tissues). Also, just as stress reduction and exercise are now known to be good for our blood vessels, such activities that improve circulation and lower stress hormones such as cortisol in the body are thought by researchers to improve the healthiness of tissues such as hair, and indeed, all of our body!

The Role of Protein in Hair Structure

Hair has unique needs and requirements of its own. Therefore it responds well to certain specific nutrients in addition to the whole backdrop of nutrients our bodies require to operate and function in an optimal manner. All nutrients are important, even vital, just as every instrument contributes to the total sound in an orchestra. But some nutrients, like some instruments, may be more prominent for certain compositions. Hair is no different.

The first thing to understand about our hair's requirements is that it is principally composed of protein.

There are many kinds of protein in the body. Hormones, such as insulin, are mostly comprised of proteins. So are the highly specialized cells and tissues that do work in our body- skeletal muscle is composed almost exclusively of protein strands. Two of the main proteins in skeletal muscle, called actin and myosin, respectively, have fascinatingly unique properties that allow muscle to do its unique job of contracting in order to move bones. Hemoglobin, the iron-containing substance in our blood that has a unique affinity for oxygen and carries it throughout the body to feed living tissues, is also a protein. And then there are the so-called "structural proteins" that give us strength and flexibility and motion- the substances that make up our connective tissues, such as our tendons, ligaments, and fascia. These tissues are made in large part of collagen and elastin, unique and strong proteins that give us strength, definition, and elasticity.

Every protein is different and unique in their composition, characteristics, and functions. What they all have in common is that they are each made of thousands of smaller units linked together into complex chains, like elaborate necklaces or rosaries. These small individual "beads" or units called "amino acids" are chemically related to each other because they almost all contain the element nitrogen, molecularly attached in specific ways.   Therefore in general, proteins are famous for being important nitrogen-containing molecules. However, there are a few key amino acids that contain another element in place of nitrogen. These amino acids use the element sulfur in place of nitrogen, and are called the "sulfur-containing amino acids". The main protein in hair, known as keratin, is a protein that is rich in these sulfur-containing amino acids.

The Role of Sulfur in Hair Health

There are only a small handful of these sulfur-containing amino acids within the human body, and each is a powerful and crucial molecular ally for health and wellbeing. Two of them, known as l-cysteine and l-methionine, are key components of healthy hair as they are incorporated into the very structure of the main protein that makes up our hair, keratin. Part of sulfur's role in making hair strong is because it participates in what are called "disulfide bonds", which serve to strengthen the protein's molecular structure-which is part of the reason why hair is (hopefully) such a strong material.

Interestingly, the strength and lightness of a bird's feathers is also due to their incorporation of keratin- with the same sulfur-containing amino acids- as ours. Sulfur supports hair growth in other ways as well. Thiamine (B_1) and Biotin, both B vitamins associated with hair growth and cell division, contain sulfur as part of their molecular structures. And sulfur is also a key component of certain enzymes, including the anti-oxidant glutathione, which protects tissues against the negative effects and attacks of excess oxygen-containing molecules known as free radicals. Such protection is also important for hair and scalp health, along with our appearance, as the oxidation of fats in the scalp is thought to be part of the process that can give rise to dry scalp and dandruff in some cases.

I call sulfur "the beauty mineral" because of its unique importance for two of the principle proteins that are keys to our health and appearance- collagen and keratin. Collagen of course, is important for the youthfulness, strength, and flexibility of skin, joint tissues, ligaments, and tendons; keratin is critical for the health of our hair, and also our skin and nails.

Sulfur is a yellow colored mineral in nature, and is the 10th most common element in the universe. And since it is crucial for the formation of essential amino acids such as taurine, cysteine and methionine, as well as the B vitamins thiamine and biotin, it is considered an essential element.

As most people know, sulfur has a strong and characteristic odor, often associated with eggs. Matches too contain sulfur, which is the other smell most commonly associated with sulfur. Another common experience many people have had encountering sulfur are at hot springs; many of the world's renowned hot springs arise from beneath sulfur-containing rock strata, and the characteristic smell of many of these springs is from the dissolved sulfur in the water. Throughout history, many of these hot springs were (and still are) renowned for their therapeutic, healing properties.

Sulfur has a long history of use as a medicinal agent, going back to ancient times. It has been used since antiquity as a natural insecticide and fungicide, and is still considered to be safe and effective for many such conditions. Many old time remedies for dandruff and other scalp conditions contained sulfur in their recipes. Even today, shampoos and other treatments for both animals and humans often contain sulfur in their formulas. Even the ancient Egyptians knew of the healing benefits of sulfur. The famous Ebers Papyrus medical document mentions sulfur treatments for skin and other disorders. In more modern times, the breakthrough discoveries of penicillin and other "sulfa" drugs revolutionized medicine's ability to treat many bacterial and fungal infections that were previously resistant to treatment.

As an essential element, it is important that sulfur be present in our diets. Good food sources of sulfur include eggs and some animal proteins. For vegetarians and vegans, sulfur is present in a number of plant- based foods. The allium family is rich in sulfur. Garlic, onions, leeks, and shallots are all sulfur- containing foods in this family. Similarly, the plant family known as the "brassicas" is also well known for its sulfur content. Cabbages (green and purple), kale, broccoli, Brussels sprouts, and cauliflower are all members of this family and can supply us with the beauty mineral, sulfur.

Another supplemental source of biologically available sulfur is MSM. MSM stands for methyl sulfonyl methane and is available as a popular, over the counter supplement. MSM is often promoted for joint and tendon health and for the repair and treatment of sprains and strains in major joint areas such as shoulders and knees. But many people are also taking it for hair and nail growth and have reported that it seems to be beneficial for them. Some reports say that MSM may aid hair growth because it might be able to lengthen the growth phase of the follcicle's cycle (called the anagen phase).

Other sulfur-containing supplements commonly used for health and beauty include glucosamine sulfate and various forms of collagen. Unfortunately, commercially sold collagen is not vegan or vegetarian-friendly, as it is derived from animal tissues. Gelatin is another animal-derived protein that contains sulfur-containing amino acids and which has been used for centuries as a support for hair and nails.

Epsom salts are another good source of sulfur. Epsom salts are a type of salt that combines magnesium and sulfur. The chemical structure of Epsom salts is called simply, "magnesium sulfate". Taken internally, Epsom salts are a strong laxative and should be used cautiously. On the other hand, Epsom salts are a wonderful additive to one's bath, and have a long history in relieving achy, tired, sore muscles from over work, exercise, etc. Of course, both sulfur as well as magnesium are essential nutrients that act beneficially on many parts of the body.

Additional Hair Nutrients

There are numerous other nutrients associated with good hair health besides sulfur and protein. Iron is important for hair development, and in some cases, severe iron deficiency (anemia) is known to be associated with hair loss. Thyroid disorders are also medically known to be a cause of hair loss, so it may be of benefit in some situations to be tested in order to rule out these medical conditions. Trace minerals, including iodine, might be of benefit for hair health, and are generally a good idea anyway for overall health and wellness. Sea vegetables, such as the sea weeds nori, kelp, hijiki, arame, wakame, dulse, kombu, and others, are good sources of both iodine as well as other trace minerals from the ocean, and might be considered as part of one's health and beauty regime.

Healthy fats are also of great importance in producing healthy hair. The omega 3's, present in walnuts, flax and chia seeds, krill, salmon, cod, and other cold water fish are thought to inhibit inflammation and support the circulatory system and flow of blood to the scalp. Inflammation can affect any tissue in the body, including scalp tissue and hair follicles. Eliminating unhealthy oils and increasing your intake of healthy oils is another key component of the 'beautiful from within' program. A healthy scalp as well as the growing hair shaft need good oils to function properly. Most of us have heard that vigorous brushing helps to bring these oils out and helps moisten and soften overly dry, brittle hair.

Two additional very important "beauty minerals" are zinc, and copper. Both are frequently found in short supply in the modern "S.A.D" (Standard American Diet) and both are important for the growth and maintenance of healthy cells. Zinc in particular is critical for new protein synthesis (creation of protein molecules out of the amino acid building blocks) so it is intimately involved in successful keratin production.

Copper is another beauty element that has not been well appreciated until recently, but it is also of vital importance in the maintenance of our health and wellbeing. Copper is a critical mineral in many pathways in our bodies. It is essential for hemoglobin synthesis (some cases of anemia are actually caused by copper deficiencies instead of iron) and it is also an essential component of the structural proteins that give us strength and elasticity- qualities associated with youthfulness, resilience, and less wrinkling. Copper also plays an important role in hair color, preventing premature graying and color loss. Copper is also a component of one of the body's main antioxidant enzymes, Super Oxide Dismutase, or SOD, and may help in dandruff control. Copper is available at good health food stores and supplement departments; not much is needed- usually 1-2 mg on a daily basis should be adequate for most adults to ensure they get all they need.

Along with copper, zinc, and sulfur, one other mineral stands out as an important "beauty nutrient". Silica, the element found in quartz and sand, is now being looked at as a key player in the "beautiful from within" arena. Silica is actually the most common element in the earth's crust, and has been incorporated into living structures since the beginning of life on earth. Silica gives bird's feathers their strength, and it is also important in keeping the stems of many plants strong and resistant. In a similar way, silica and what are known as silicate compounds, might give added strength and flexibility to tissues such as hair, nails, and skin.

Besides minerals such as silica, sulfur, zinc, and copper, some of the vitamins are also crucial for healthy hair development and growth. Two of the B vitamins, Biotin and Folic Acid, are strongly associated with hair health. Folic acid is an important molecule that helps cells divide in a healthy way, and has long been thought to help prevent the premature graying of hair. It is also a vital nutrient for many other reasons, and is known to prevent certain forms of anemia, and may even help with fatigue and apathy in some individuals. Another B vitamin, pantothenic acid (sometimes known as B_5) is also associated with helping delay gray hair onset. The other B vitamin associated with healthy hair is Biotin. Vegans may not get enough of this essential vitamin, as it is mainly found in relative abundance in eggs, liver, and other animal products. One study, coming out of Harvard, concluded that biotin is "one of the most important nutrients for preserving hair strength, texture, and function."

Like our skin, hair is an external tissue, meaning it is constantly exposed to the stresses and challenges of our environment. Having healthy hair takes attention, and a pro-active approach. Harsh chemicals, chlorine, too much sun, overly hot blow dryers and many hair care treatments can all stress our hair and challenge our best attempts to grow it long and beautiful and healthy. So too does everyday stress; chronic stress activates our sympathetic nervous system- the famous "fight or flight" syndrome, which can elevate our cortisol levels. Cortisol, a common stress hormone, is thought to adversely affect hair growth by inhibiting the growth phase of the follicles. In fact many people have reported that their hair has literally fallen out due to extreme, prolonged stress. For real health and beauty, counteracting stress through whatever means can be a vitally important remedy. Whether that means frequent hot baths, quietly listening to soothing music, getting a massage, doing yoga, taking walks in the park or getting out in nature- and in general giving ourselves permission to unwind- all can have a positive impact on our body's beauty tissues, especially our skin and hair.

With our understanding of the principles of "Beautiful from Within"- that we are what we eat- and that beauty comes from within- we can realize that the means to looking our best from our head down to our toes is literally in our hands. Avoiding the bad things- smoking, stress, harsh environmental chemicals and conditions, too much alcohol, and depriving our body of the nutrients it needs- are all important measures that everyone can take. Scientists and researchers know that starvation, caloric deprivation, inadequate protein intake, not enough essential fatty acids, and less than optimal trace mineral consumption can all result in poor hair growth and quality. Ensuring that your diet contains optimal amounts of these by being more nutrient-dense is clearly the key to having the head of hair you want- and deserve.

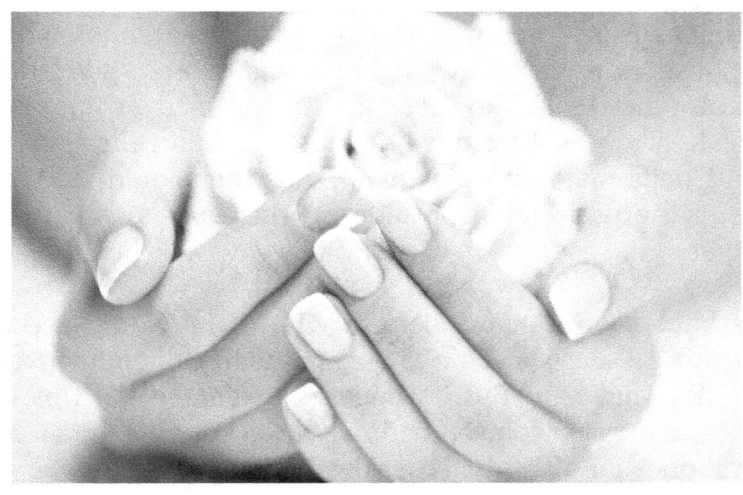

Chapter 6

Hard as Nails

Nails adorn our fingers and toes, and all twenty of these hard tissues allow us to grip, tear, scratch, and hold. They also are one of the most decorated parts of the human body. Our nails are definitely one of our body's premier "beauty tissues" and we spend literally countless hundreds of millions of dollars on them every year- polishing, decorating, and mani/pedi curing them.

Nails are the human version of many animal's claws. Strangely they are also closely related in their composition to hair- and horns. Both hair and nails (and horns) are composed principally of protein, and both share the same protein as their major constituent- keratin. Keratin gives tissues their special hardness and strength, imparting to them the specialized functions they need for protecting the body from danger, accidents, or abuse.

Polishing nails is a custom that dates way back in human history. Nail polish can certainly highlight nails and give them a dramatic, fancy look. And it can also serve to cover up nails that are weak, brittle, split, ridged or blotchy. All of these are signs that our nails may not be as healthy as they could be. We may cover up the underlying problem in this way- but it certainly won't get to the root cause of poor nail growth or health.

As we have seen, "beautiful from within" nutrition has a very significant, even crucial role to play in the health and appearance of our skin and hair. But its benefits extend to the tips of our fingers and toes as well! Nutrition plays a key role in nail health, just as it does for all of the other tissues in our body.

It is no secret that nails are one of the harder tissues in our bodies. Teeth, bones, and nails are all really tough, hard tissues. Teeth and bones are primarily a mixture of phosphorus and calcium salts in association with some proteins. Nails, along with hair, by contrast, are mostly proteins; and a unique one in particular- keratin.

Obviously nails and hair are not the same. Externally they are structurally and functionally quite different tissues altogether. But they do share a similar chemical and molecular make-up. As we learned in the section on hair, keratin is a rather unique protein molecule in that it has a strong sulfur component in it. That is because two of the principle amino acids in the keratin protein molecule are L-cysteine and L-methionine, both sulfur-containing amino acids. Sulfur amino acids form extraordinarily strong bonds, giving them their characteristic strength and rigidity- perfect for making strong tissues like hair fibers and nail plates. In nails the keratin is "glued" together, like a laminated wood board. Such layering imparts much of the strength to our nails, and allows them to be the specialized body parts that we need, such as for peeling an orange, or gripping on to something (or somebody). Surprisingly, calcium is not that much of a factor in contributing to nail hardness, like we find in bones and the skeleton. However, minerals do play a role, and it is true that calcium- along with other minerals such as magnesium, iron, zinc, sodium, and copper- are all present in nails and contribute to the total picture of nail health.

In general nails are primarily protein by composition, and protein-deficient diets, along with general malnourishment definitely can lead to weakened, brittle, or misshaped nails. Malnourishment can be caused by a wide variety of situations, from chronic alcoholism to anorexia and other eating disorders to poverty, to drug and medication induced mal-absorption or faulty metabolism. In addition, a wide range of unrelated conditions, from chronic stress to medications to cigarette smoking, can lead to a reduction in stomach acid secretion, which can ultimately also interfere with protein digestion and amino acid absorption.

Besides inadequate or insufficient protein, other nutrients can also influence the appearance and health of our nails. Zinc deficiencies can result in white spots under the nail bed, while a darkened curved end may be due to a B_{12} deficiency. Brittle and weak nails may be due to either inadequate calcium or vitamin A. Iron deficiency-associated anemia is well known to be a cause of brittle nails that are prone to longitudinal splitting. Anorexia, as mentioned above, not only can lead to brittle nails, but also to longitudinal splitting or peeling of the nail tissue. And chronic low magnesium intake may result in soft, flaky nails that are prone to splitting or breaking easily.

It can be difficult sometimes to pinpoint exactly which nutrient in short supply is contributing to nail problems. But to be on the safe side, a good general program for optimal nail health would be sure to include plenty of protein (especially proteins containing the sulfur amino acids Cysteine and Methionine), the B vitamin Biotin, essential fatty acids, vitamin C, B6, iron, vitamin D, and silica. Silica is the principle mineral found in sand, and is the most abundant mineral in the earth's crust. This humble mineral is suspected to be useful in strengthening tissues such as hair and nails in humans, in the same way that it does for feathers, scales, and other structures in the rest of the animal kingdom. Many silica supplements are now on the market and are well worth trying. (It beats eating sand!)

Beautifully painted nails can be a fun form of self-expression, celebration, and indulgence. But ideally your fingernails and toenails should be a healthy canvas for that splash of color at the ends of your extremities. Radiant health- and being "beautiful from within" really should encompass and cover your entire body- all the way to the very tips of your fingers and toes.

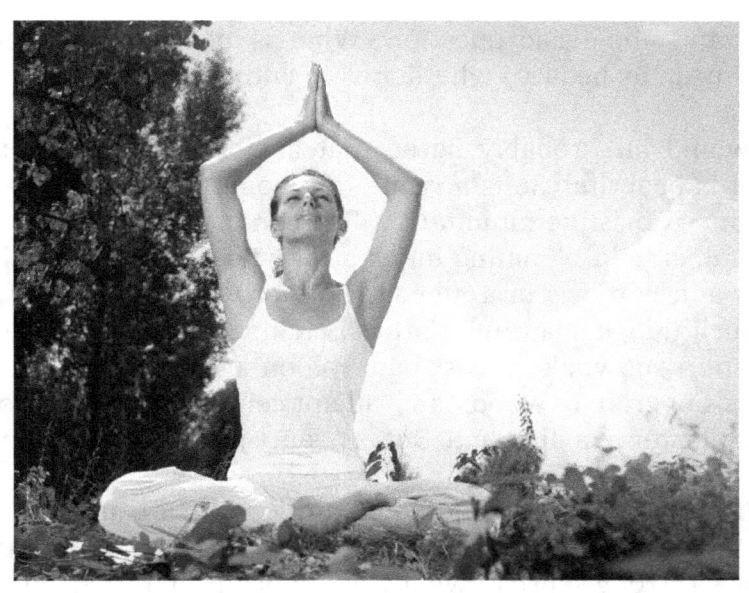

Chapter 7

Holistic Beauty:
Living the Beautiful Life

So far in this book I have tried to show you the many ways with which you can take a proactive stance with respect to working with and protecting and enhancing your beauty assets-specifically the outer tissues of your hair, skin, and nails.

We have looked at some of the external threats and challenges to your body as well as the inner nutritional needs and requirements necessary to preserve, protect, and enhance your cellular health. By now you should feel empowered through the knowledge of what foods and supplements can offer help, and what foods and substances to avoid. But all of this begs an important, and basic question: What is beauty? What do we really mean by beauty –whether from within or without.

We would all probably agree that a vibrant red and orange sunset is beautiful. So is a rising full moon, coming up over the horizon. A pristine mountain valley complete with a cascading waterfall, a field blooming in a riot of wild flowers, the brilliant colors and patterns of a monarch butterfly's wing- most would find such things beautiful. Nature is full to bursting with objects of beauty- snowflakes, frost patterns on a window, the swirling patterns of grain in wood, the brilliant colors of a rainbow or the shining luster in a diamond. But is beauty just a physical thing?

Certainly most of us find the natural world beautiful. Many objects and creations of art are a bit more subjective, but most of us have a strong sense of what we find beautiful in art, paintings, sculpture, textiles and architecture. And most of the time people can agree on a beautiful person as well. But it is also true that different cultures and times can have vastly different concepts of what is considered "beautiful".

Beauty can be physical, but non-physical beauty, as in a moving piece of music or a voice lifted in song- can also be beautiful. The shape of a mouth, a nose, one's lips, or cheekbones- all can be seen as beautiful, and so of course can the orchestrated coordination of each part composed together into a face. A young woman or man may be beautiful, but so too can an octogenarian- with beauty, wisdom, and kindness etched into their face, with character, humility, humor, wisdom, compassion, and other attributes shining through.

But what else do we mean when we refer to "beauty"? The shape of one's eyes, or lips might be considered "beautiful" or attractive, but is it the shape alone, or color, or lash length that is beautiful, or is it perhaps some underlying quality? Perhaps beauty is not so much about shapes, sizes, and proportions, as it is about vitality, clarity, radiance, healthiness, and joyfulness. This book is about all kinds of beauty- both outer, physical beauty of course- our hair, skin, and nails- but it is also about health, radiance, and vitality- the kinds of energetic beauty that anyone can achieve, at any age, under any circumstances.

Beautiful from Within is your guide to healthy skin, hair, and nails- but it is also a book about how to achieve your potential- your health, vitality and energy: all key aspects of your "total beauty package".

Beauty truly shines from within, and the sparkle in one's eyes, an alert curious enjoyment of life, a sense of humor and fairness, the empathy of truly listening- and caring- about another- all of these are also forms of beauty, even if less tangible and sometimes less honored by our culture, which often seems to elevate youthfulness above all else.

Beauty is many things, but above all I would say that *beauty is life,* and life is beautiful- and it is precious. In other words, we are all- each one of us- beautiful, and worthy beings. This may sound obvious, but in today's competitive, fast paced, always busy world, some of us may forget our own beauty, and the gifts we bring to the world just by being here. Celebrating who we are as truly unique individuals- this is an important message that we risk forgetting if we don't sometimes pause from the hustle and bustle of our fast paced, perpetually plugged in 21st century lives and give ourselves permission to take quality "time out".

The old expression, "take time to stop and smell the roses" means to give oneself permission to pause, slow down, reflect, and *be present* with the moment. We may forget at times that *each moment* is precious, and in so doing, squander some of our precious lives in stress, anxiety, worry, and fear. Being beautiful from within has many meanings- and one of them is that our inner beauty comes from having beautiful thoughts, beautiful feelings, beautiful emotions. Tension, stress, worry, fear- all play out in our faces, in our eyes, and in our skin. The good news is that so too does contentment, acceptance, joy in the happiness of others, compassion, and love.

You are special. Sometimes every one of us can forget this amidst the challenges and hurdles of life. Yet the simple remembrance of our own special uniqueness is perhaps the biggest key to unlocking the treasures of beauty that lie within us.

Several times in this book the stress hormone, cortisol has been mentioned. Secreted by the adrenal glands in response to stress of different kinds, elevated cortisol is associated with all manner of health problems, including lowered resistance to disease, lowered immunity, poor wound healing, thinner, more fragile skin, and accelerated aging.

The central theme of *"Beautiful from Within"* is learning how to take better care of yourself. In addition to eating right, taking the appropriate supplements, and avoiding counterproductive lifestyle patterns and habits such as smoking, drinking, and eating junk food, we need to also learn how to unwind, relax, and give ourselves permission to sometimes "just be". Lowering our stress level (and stress hormones such as cortisol) is critical to looking – and feeling- our best.

I call this approach your "holistic beauty" strategy. Holistic beauty techniques encompass a wide spectrum of stress reduction and supportive approaches that provide us with energy, reduce stress, and refresh and rejuvenate us on all levels. They represent the "permission" we need to give ourselves the space to take time out for ourselves if we are to truly look and feel our best. Having fun, remembering to laugh at life (and at ourselves) is a big- and too often forgotten- side of life that we all deserve to take part in.

Yoga, hot baths, walks in the park, time out with best friends, playing with and appreciating pets and other animals, sitting quietly in meditation and prayer, making art, gardening, star gazing, going to a concert or museum, volunteering or giving time to a charity or helping those in need, listening to a friend or child with a non- judgmental, open heart- these are just some of the many ways we can restore, rejuvenate, and refresh ourselves- and I'm sure you can come up with many others of your own!

The bottom line is that you are worth taking care of. When we value ourselves equally with others, and find our hearts open to the beauty of the world, then we can truly find the beauty within- and everywhere.

Why Stress is Anti-Beauty...
(...and what to do about it!)

No one likes to feel stressed out. Stress is....well, stressful, and is the direct result of pressure, deadlines, worry, bills, bad news, poor health, break-ups, bad bosses (or bad employees), and a zillion other causes. Stress *feels* crummy. But it also affects how we look as well.

Stress is not just "all in your head." Actually stress is in your body- specifically, in your bloodstream. Stress is actually related to the circulation in the body of a specific hormone, called cortisol. Cortisol is secreted from the adrenal glands, which sit in your lower back, just on top of the kidneys. Stress can be sudden, such as when you have to slam on your brakes because the person in the car who was texting and driving almost hit you, or it can be long-term, or "chronic".

Sudden stress can be lifesaving, because it helps you react quickly and can give you a quick burst of energy which can help you deal with an emergency or threat. On the other hand, chronic, relatively low level stress can be quite debilitating, and can have cumulative long term negative consequences on your body, mind, health, and looks.

What you need to know about stress and cortisol is how to lower it, what raises it, and why it can affect your health and appearance. With this information, hopefully you will be motivated to take the important, necessary, and useful steps to help control your stress levels.

What are some of the negative effects of stress? Researchers and doctors have long known that the effects are many and varied. Some of the documented effects of chronic stress include anxiety, depression, sleep disorders, weight gain (particularly abdominal or "belly fat"), memory lapses, thyroid disorders, sugar imbalances, decreased libido (sex drive), decreased or slow wound healing, hair loss, and a loss in muscle mass. Recognize any of these symptoms in yourself?

Chronically elevated cortisol levels inhibit protein synthesis and in particular the production by our body of collagen. One published scientific study says that cortisol-induced collagen loss was TEN TIMES GREATER IN THE SKIN than in any other tissue! When collagen is lost from the skin, the result is wrinkling and sagging, less firm, less elastic skin. Cortisol hurts our collagen levels in two ways- by both hastening the breakdown of this vital "beauty molecule" and by inhibiting the creation of fresh collagen in the body. Double whammy!

Fortunately we can do a lot to reduce cortisol levels and its negative effects. Since cortisol is produced by our adrenal glands in response to stress, the key is to lower our stress levels and to learn how to better deal or cope with stress in our lives. Here are some quick suggestions- all of the following have been shown scientifically to help reduce cortisol levels: massage, deep breathing, music, laughter, exercise, sex/intimacy, conversation, sunshine, yoga, hot baths, visualization, meditation, participating in hobbies, community events, prayer. And the list goes on.

We are what we eat. Food can certainly raise- or lower- cortisol levels. Excess caffeine, too much sugar, processed fats, too much sodium, even too much meat (it contains elevated levels of stress hormones such as adrenaline and cortisol from the fear in the animals about to be slaughtered)- all can raise our cortisol levels. On the other hand, certain foods can lower cortisol and help make it more manageable. Foods rich in vitamin C and B vitamins have been shown to be very helpful. Similarly, foods that are nutrient-dense for magnesium (a relaxing and calming mineral) such as green vegetables and leafy greens like kale, spinach, chard, bok choy, and many others) can be very helpful. Green tea contains a useful substance, called L-theanine, which is also an effective anti-stress substance. Other relaxing and soothing herbs, like chamomile can be helpful too. Tulsi, a tea made from a plant known as holy basil, is a wonderful adaptogen, or stress adapter. Other ways to help combat stress include taking omega 3 fatty acids and enjoying small amounts of dark chocolate or even a little organic red wine!

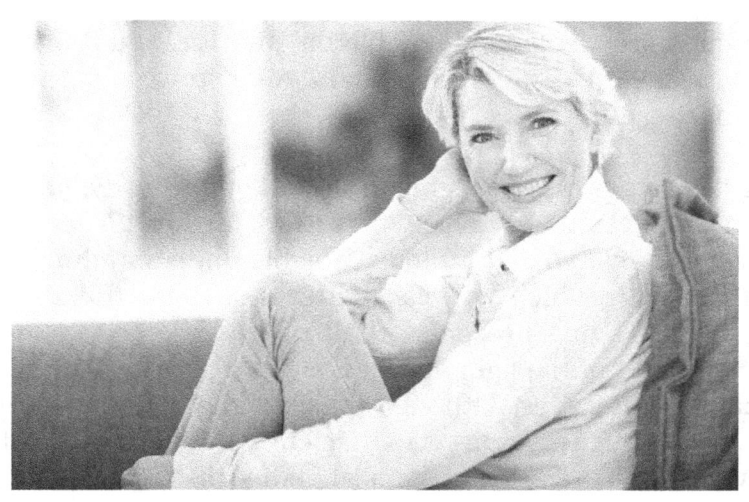

Chapter 8

Growing Gracefully from Within

As we travel through the personal journey that we call "our life" we accumulate many things—experiences, memories, friends, lessons. We become "wiser" as we mature: typically we become more understanding, more patient, more easy-going. We may learn that it is not worth it "to sweat the small stuff"- and sometimes we can even see that "it is all small stuff," at least relatively speaking.

Life certainly can be stressful at times, but hopefully we learn from our mistakes and hopefully we also learn to roll with the punches that life inevitably brings our way. We also learn little by little to not always take ourselves so seriously. All of these lessons and tests are simply part of the ride- and hopefully for the most part, it is an interesting and relatively joyous one.

But bumps are virtually inevitable on any ride, and it is how we deal with them that defines us and demonstrates our character and inner resources.

Aging is a fact of life. But aging is also an opportunity, like all the other challenges that we face in our life. Ideally *"Beautiful from Within"* will give you additional, valuable understanding, insight and tools with which you can better deal with the inevitable changes that aging presents to all of us and our bodies. Our understanding of the aging process has progressed rapidly over the past few decades. Although much of the story is still being worked out in the details, most scientists feel fairly confident that we now have a pretty good handle on much of the story behind the aging process. And much of this story is now being played out in health food stores, vitamin aisles, and grocery store shelves.

By now, virtually everyone has heard of anti-oxidants. In foods, supplements, cosmetics—anti-oxidants are everywhere. In this book, too, we have discussed the importance of anti-oxidants— from ascorbic acid to zinc, anti-oxidants are crucial allies in the *"Beautiful from Within"* system. But why?

As the word implies, anti-oxidants work against oxygen— protecting us from it. Of course, we all know that oxygen is vital to life on earth; it is absolutely essential for our survival. But too much oxygen— like too much of the sun's rays— can sometimes be detrimental to our bodies. Oxygen, along with certain other molecules, can turn into more dangerous forms that are called "free-radicals." And the danger of these free-radicals is that they are aggressive molecular renegades that attack and damage healthy, normal tissues.
Free-radicals accelerate aging by damaging cells and tissues that may not regain their original, fresh state. Wrinkled skin, dry arthritic joint tissue, loss of hair color, and even the pigments

that are sometimes deposited in our skin and are known as "liver spots" (or age spots) are all signs of free-radical damage.
So are cataracts, and so are many other age-related symptoms. Even the inflammation and damage to the skin associated with a severe sunburn is another example of the effects of free-radicals generated by the ultraviolet rays interacting with molecules in the skin.

Most symptoms of free-radical damage are slowly accumulated and therefore often go unnoticed until they become too obvious to ignore. But much of the emerging science of nutrition is about addressing the issue of free-radicals— how they form, what contributes to them, and how to slow down or neutralize their negative effects.

While much remains to be understood, we have come a long way in understanding the science behind free-radicals and the anti-oxidant molecules that are our defense against them. Let's briefly examine this situation now so we can put some of our understanding to good use.

Scientists call the damage that oxygen "species" of free-radicals cause: "oxidative stress." Oxidative stress simply refers to the pressure, stress, or damage that these molecules cause to living systems. We refer to different "species" of free-radicals simply because there are dozens or more of these molecules —each one slightly different in how it works, what generates it, and how common it is.

We have known for many years of the dangers associated with cigarette smoking. Cigarettes generate "tars"— sticky glue-like material that comes from the charred and burnt residues of the tobacco itself. And tar literally does act like glue; it sticks to and slows down the function of cilia— tiny, hair-like structures that line the respiratory tree and normally help to sweep debris and other unwanted particles away. Tar can also "gum up" or clog and impede the transfer of oxygen from the air we breathe into the red blood cells that ultimately carry oxygen to all of the cells of our body.

But cigarettes are nasty in other respects as well. In addition to tar and nicotine, burning organic compounds (there are literally hundreds of added compounds in most commercial brands of tobacco) generates free radicals— in huge amounts. In fact, it is estimated that each inhalation of cigarette smoke brings billions of these free radical molecules directly into the bloodstream of the smoker (and huge amounts in the "second-hand smoke" that nearby co-workers and other bystanders inhale as well).

This is a main reason why it is said that each cigarette destroys from 30 to 50 mg of vitamin C (ascorbic acid). It might be more accurate to say it this way: each cigarette requires up to 50 mg of vitamin C that is (hopefully) present in the body to defend it from the damaging and toxic effects of the free radicals from each cigarette. So if you smoke, vitamin C is recruited from within your body to neutralize these radical molecules. And if not destroyed, these radicals are available to attack vulnerable molecules in our skin, eyes, blood vessels, and brain— leading to inflammation or damage that inevitably causes those tissues to age and not look or function quite as well as they originally did.

Smokers who inhale, say, ten cigarettes a day therefore require at least an additional 500 mg of vitamin C a day, just to break even compared to non-smokers.

Cigarettes are probably one of the most famous and obvious causes of accelerated aging and disease. But there are some other common environmental or dietary hazards that we are exposed to as well. Several have already been mentioned in the pages of this book, but it might be beneficial to repeat them here for emphasis.

Alcohol can be a potent generator of free radicals. Many of us have seen the effects first hand in loved ones or friends of the ravaging effects of alcohol misuse or abuse. In addition to the social and personal miseries alcoholism can lead to, accelerated aging from excessive drinking is another.

Certain alcoholic drinks can be worse than others in this regard. Whereas some are quite nasty, a few might actually be neutral or relatively good for us. Some research, for example, indicates that red wine when consumed moderately can actually offer some useful anti-oxidant protection. This might be due to some of the compounds that originate in the grape's purple skin—pigments called polyphenols, such as resveratrol. In fact, a lot of anti-aging research on resveratrol has supported the hypothesis that this substance is actually quite beneficial for skin and arterial health. And yes, this seems to indicate that it is red wine, not white, that is the healthier option. In addition to being in red wine, resveratrol is present in grape juice and many other foods, and is now available in supplement form in capsules.

The other "relatively" healthier alcohol options, in my opinion, are some of the "microbrew" beers. Because many of these are unpasteurized "live" fermented beverages, the enzymes and some of the B vitamins present have not been destroyed by the high heat of pasteurization. Therefore, I consider those beers, like red wine, to be relatively nutrient-dense and acceptable when one wants to responsibly have some alcohol for social or celebratory reasons.

What then are the unhealthiest alcoholic drinks? It turns out that the spirits that have been heavily distilled may be the worst. Distilling alcohol, and concentrating it, seems to generate a very potent class of molecular radicals called "urethanes". Similar to the polyurethane varnishes often used to waterproof and treat wood flooring or cabinets, urethanes are considered incredibly toxic to the liver and other tissues. Brandy, whiskey, bourbon, sherry, and other strong spirits are often heavily contaminated with high urethane levels. I strongly urge anyone who cares about their health and looks to avoid these!

In addition to the obvious toxic contributions of cigarettes and hard alcohol, there are many less obvious sources of free radicals in our environment and foods. Unfortunately, they are surprisingly common. Normally consumed in small amounts, nonetheless their danger might lie in the constant small insults and challenging "oxidative stresses" that can inevitably add up. In the same way, avoiding these by "erring on the side of caution" and taking small pro-active steps might lead to a healthier, longer, and hopefully more disease-free life.

One extremely common and perhaps surprising source of free-radicals is the pesticides and other synthetic food additives found in non-organic foods. Pesticides often work their destruction on insects and other pests by the actions of their free radicals on the nervous systems or respiration of their victims. Small amounts of pesticides in our produce can add up over a lifetime of exposure. Certified organic produce might offer long-term lower risks to us by reducing our overall exposure or "toxic load."

Similarly, hydrogenated oils (or "trans-fats") are molecularly altered from their natural states and might contribute radicals to the diet. Certainly, the altered shapes of these synthetic, modified fats are now known to accelerate aging by damaging cellular membranes when they are incorporated into cells and tissues instead of being metabolized for energy the way most lipids are. This is another example of "you are what you eat."

Eating damaged, altered fats is simply not a good way to protect or optimize yourself. Fried foods, too, are generators of radicals; highly heated fats and oils are very unhealthy and should be avoided whenever possible for the best possible "beauty from within" outcome.

Refined sugars, too, are associated with accelerated aging. Where their action in accelerating aging might not be directly due so much to free radicals, the chemical reactions that such sugars are known to participate in by attaching themselves to key proteins is equally damaging. Known as a "glycation" process to scientists, heating sugars in the presence of a protein creates a sticky situation where the protein is actually altered or damaged by the "hitchhiking" attached sugar.

Such "advanced glycation end products" (or AGES for short) are strongly linked with damaged, aged tissues. AGES are prevalent in cataracts, skin aging, and the plaques in the brain that are found in certain diseases such as Parkinson's and some dementias. Poorly controlled blood sugar, such as in some forms of hypoglycemia , adult-onset diabetes, or the condition known as "syndrome X," might accelerate aging and some disease onsets through this mechanism of glycating proteins— sometimes referred to as "cross linked" proteins. Cross-linked proteins can make our cells stiffer, less pliable, and more subject to damage and premature aging. Watching and limiting our intake of refined sugars is an important and smart long-term strategy in the "beautiful from within" program. High fructose corn syrup is also known to increase the propensity for glycation to occur.

We mentioned vitamin C (ascorbic acid) in regard to helping protect against some of these free-radicals. But Vitamin C is only one form of protection. Ascorbic acid is water soluble— so it offers protection within the tissues and components of your body that are water-based. But there are many tissues in your body that are not water-based or soluble. These other tissues are lipid or fat-based tissues. And they need protection just as badly as the others.

Fortunately, there are forms of anti-oxidants that are lipid-soluble. Whereas vitamin C is the most famous water-soluble anti-oxidant, vitamin E is probably the most famous lipid or fat-soluble anti-oxidant. Numerous studies have shown its effectiveness, too, in offering protection for the many fat-soluble cellular structures in the body. There are many forms of vitamin E on the market, but I strongly encourage you to seek out a natural form of the vitamin. Most of the cheaper vitamin E out there is a synthetic version, which may not be nearly as effective. Check with a knowledgeable person at your health food store. It is worth it to pay more and get the right stuff! As far as food sources go, vitamin E is present in almonds, sunflower and other seeds and nuts, avocados, and spinach. If fresh and unprocessed, all of these foods could be considered ideal in the "beautiful from within" program.

There are many great foods and supplements available that should be considered for any good anti-aging program, which generally offer us additional protection and benefits. This is the basis of the nutrient-dense, Nude food approach—anti-oxidant-rich, nutrient-rich, unprocessed, natural, colorful, fresh foods, that supply us with vitamins, minerals, pigments and enzymes should be the focus of our diets. This is why we emphasize diverse foods— a good variety of foods from around the world gives our bodies a nice variety of protective molecules that can act in different ways to offer protection in a variety of ways.

Antioxidant-rich, Nude foods include such diverse foods as blueberries, pomegranates, kiwi fruit, dark chocolate, green teas, and turmeric. Baby greens, sprouts, fresh flax oil, fresh juices such as a carrot/veggie juice blend, and many others can all offer protective benefits and work their magic in helping slow down the aging process. But remember, this is a two-step process. Lots of the "good stuff"—the super foods and herbs and supplements we have been talking about— that is step one. But equally important is the other step— eliminating the "bad stuff." And now you know exactly what I mean by the bad stuff: hard alcohol, tobacco, refined sugars, fried and bad fats and oils, empty calories, low-fiber foods, and hormone (and cruelty) containing animal products. Do the good stuff, cut out the bad, and find plenty of quality time for lowering stress and anxiety, and you have a great prescription for slowing down aging and raising the overall quality of your life.

Life is short and tends to pass too quickly for most of us. Extracting the maximum quality out of each day, living with gratitude and joy, and spreading happiness to those around us— these are the attributes of what I call "living a graceful and beautiful life." And it is available to each and every one of us.

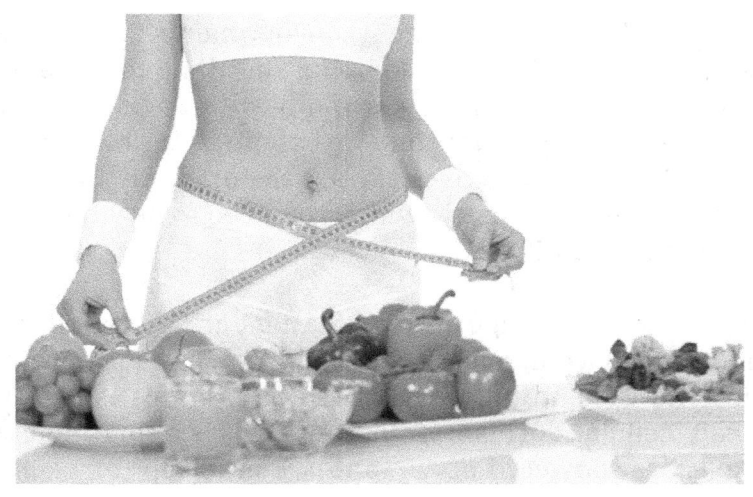

Chapter 9

The Beauty of Weight Loss from Within

The same principles of Beautiful From Within apply for weight loss as much as they do for hair, skin, and nails. Being beautiful from within means being healthy from within. And being your appropriate weight is also a reflection of your inner state of health as well.

Your inner health is another way of saying your "metabolism", and the health of your metabolism is essential to whether you easily gain weight or burn calories and find it hard to put on weight.

You have learned that "beautiful from within" comes from being well nourished within and you have also learned that a nutrient-dense diet is the best way to nourish your hair, skin, and nails as well as your overall health. The important thing to remember is that nourishing every cell of your body with the right vitamins, minerals, and other nutrients is essential to having active, healthy cells. Healthy, active cells are the only way to be able to convert calories into energy- which you need to be vital, creative, energetic, and beautiful.

When your cells are sluggish, or inefficient at converting calories to energy, then your energy levels do down, and more of the calories you eat end up being stored as fat. This is a situation that I call "cellular dormancy". Basically this is a condition where your cells are "powered down" and are in "sleep" or rest mode. Such a condition is characterized by energy storage (in the form of fat) rather than energy production.

Cells "normally" do a good job of converting food into energy. But in order to do this, they need plenty of nutrients- vitamins and minerals- for the biochemical chain reactions to occur. This complicated process occurs in the "energy factories" within your cells called mitochondria. And for your mitochondria to do a good, efficient job at producing energy, vital nutrients such as B vitamins and other factors need to be present.

This is where a nutrient-dense diet comes in. If your diet is largely S.A.D., then you are trying to feed your cells with a lot of empty calories. And as you know now, empty calories are calories that simply do not have the required B vitamins, minerals and other nutrients in adequate amounts to drive these biochemical reactions forward. As a result of being deprived of enough nutrients, your cells have no choice but to power down. The result? Everything you eat "turns to fat".

Fortunately the solution to this dilemma is pretty simple. Instead of eating a lot of empty-calorie "junk" foods, you need to make the switch- to nutrient-dense calories and foods.

What nutrients are most needed in order for our cells to hum along efficiently, burning calories and doing their jobs? The answer is clear when we look at the actual process of generating energy- the biochemical chain reactions that scientists call "the Krebs cycle".

Without going too deeply into the complicated biochemistry of producing energy, let's summarize the process by looking at the starting point and the end result. The starting point for energy production (most of the time) are carbohydrate molecules. Generally what happens is that starches or sugars get broken down until they become what is called "pyruvate". Pyruvate, or pyruvic acid, can be thought of like pieces of coal or chips of wood that are thrown into the furnace or fireplace to be burned to give us heat. But sugars are not the only sources of fuel for energy production. Fats and even proteins can be called upon for energy when the need arises.

In order for the mitochondria to be able to turn sugars, fats, and occasionally amino acids into energy, many conditions have to come together within the mitochondria where the Kreb's cycle takes place. In particular the B vitamins- Thiamine, riboflavin, and niacin need to be present. In addition carnitine, an amino acid like molecule is necessary as a transporter of simple fat structures. Finally, additional nutrients like Co Q10 and ribose need to be present as well.

The other key factor that is of great importance is the health of the cell and mitochondrial membranes. This is one of the big reasons why the nutrient-dense diet and the "beautiful from within" program both emphasize healthy fats and oils (collectively called, "lipids"). Healthy membranes allow nutrients to more easily cross over and into the cell where they can "contribute to the cause". This is also another important reason why fried, damaged, and altered fats can "gum up the works" and slow down our metabolism by interfering with cellular membranes and their properties. Fried foods don't really make you fat because of their caloric content-rather they are harmful because they make it harder for our cells to do their jobs!

Weight loss is a complicated subject involving many factors. Lifestyle, genetics, metabolism-interfering drugs and other things can all contribute to a body that is out of balance, metabolically challenged, and overweight. Yet a nourishing nutrient-dense diet can do a lot to help "unlock" a stuck metabolic situation and help you get back on track again! My book, "The Nutrient-Dense Diet" (published by Organic Healthy Living) contains a lot more information on this important subject.

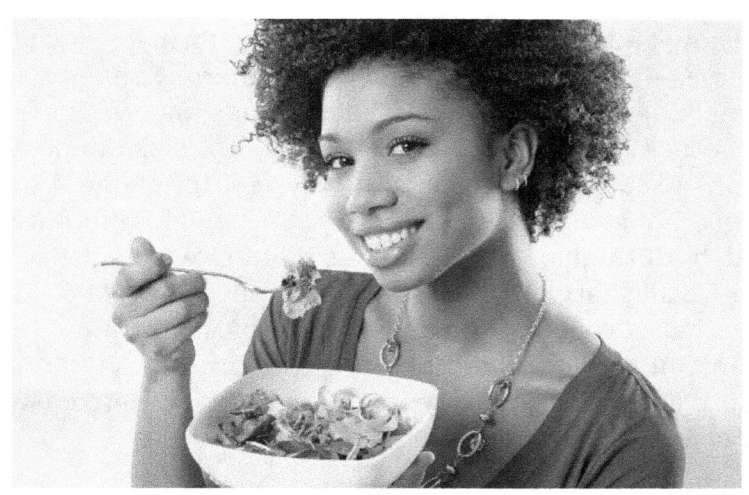

Chapter 10

Summary of the *Beautiful from Within* Program

The *Beautiful from Within* program is a combination of scientific facts and knowledge about nutrition and its many roles and functions in the body, joined with common sense. Yet, sometimes "common sense isn't all that common" anymore. Nonetheless, I believe in the basic goodness, intelligence and intuition of most people. I really believe that given the right information and support, most people are quite capable of changing for the better, making new choices, and exercising options for self-improvement. And I believe that *most* of the time, most of us do have an abundance of "common sense".

Food- how and what we eat- is a struggle for many, a challenge for some, a joyous opportunity for others. Some of us are extremely open-minded towards new foods and ways of eating, while others among us are much more close-minded and resistant to making changes and may feel intimidated or a bit frightened of even trying new things. We are all different in this regard, but I think one of the things that unite us is the common desire we all share to be healthy and happy. How we go about it is as varied as we are. But humans are typically inspired by hope and most of us have a decent streak of optimism within us. We all know deep down that tomorrow *could* be a better day than today or yesterday.

I know that most of the readers of *Beautiful from Within* probably have a fairly limited background in biochemistry, cell physiology, medical science, or clinical nutrition. Fortunately that doesn't really matter much in terms of your becoming better informed and more empowered regarding your eating choices and how you choose to nourish and support yourself. The common sense I referred to above really boils down to trusting your intuition. As adults we have all "been around the block" enough times to draw some fairly obvious conclusions about life and our world in general, and our bodies in particular. Nutrition isn't really about holding on to a particular political point of view or outlook either. When I call it "common sense" I mean that learning how to nourish ourselves is something accessible to everyone- not just professors, researchers, or doctors.

Food- shopping for it, cooking it, growing it, and eating it- is in our DNA. It is part of our inherited wisdom- our ancestral wisdom- that has been handed down for untold numbers of generations of humans. Good food nourishes us- and good food- "nutrient-dense food" is exactly what supports and fosters us- and gives us the "beauty from within" that we all crave and know we deserve.

The foundation of *Beautiful From Within* is food. As I stated on the very first page, "we are what we eat"- and this is literally true for every molecule, cell, tissue, and organ in your body. *Ideally* we should be able to get all the nutrients we need from our diets. However, the reality for most of us is that our diets will probably not be able to fulfill that lofty goal all of the time. Depleted soils, idiosyncratic personal eating habits, inherited food sensitivities, and the realities of dining in 21st century America with its agricultural system that cuts corners whenever possible and adds all manner of synthetic and artificial food additives make such an ideal difficult, if not impossible.

Still our "food matters"- as much, if not more than ever. I think that given the realities, stresses, and pressures of modern life, it is of the utmost importance that we eat with care, mindfulness, attention, and awareness. Self-respect requires it. Concern for the world- the environment- demands it. And our health, well-being, and looks- deserve it.

In the previous pages I have mentioned a number of foods that support our bodies in general and our "beauty tissues"- our hair, skin, and nails- in particular. Specifically mentioned for example were sulfur sources such as are found in foods as diverse as eggs, broccoli, garlic, and onions. As well, we talked about the importance of "nude" foods in general; foods that are nutrient-dense for various anti-oxidants, pigments, enzymes, amino acids, essential oils and fats, fiber, vitamins, and minerals. These nude foods are the good foods that I mention when I talk about the "goodness of good foods". And these of course are really the heart and soul of the *Beautiful from Within* approach to looking and feeling our best.

In this chapter, I want to highlight, repeat, and emphasize the various aspects of the *Beauty from Within* program for total health and well-being. I also want to make sure that you, the reader, see the ways these components interrelate and reinforce one another. *Integrating* into your life these various ideas and habits is the best way to truly create an effective approach to taking charge of your life, and most importantly, of getting the results you desire and deserve.

Summary of the program

Diet

1. **Drink plenty of pure water.** Preferably without chlorine or fluoride!

2. **Eat nude.** Incorporate nutrient-dense food choices whenever and wherever possible.

3. **Eat naturally colorful foods-** bright, vibrant foods are generally fresh, alive, and usually unprocessed. Salads and fruits are fun, healthy, delicious, and full of fiber and free-radical fighting anti-oxidants from their colorful pigments.

4. **Eat lots of raw "live" foods.** I am not saying you have to become a 100% "raw foodist". But I do strongly believe that incorporating larger amounts of raw/live foods is a generally smart and beneficial thing to do. Since "you are what you eat", it follows that eating lots of live/raw foods just might contribute to 'livening up' your metabolism and energy levels. I have yet to find an overweight, sluggish, depressed, live food advocate!

5. **Fresh juices.** This is really an extension of #1, 2, and 3. Juicing is a fabulous way to get concentrated levels of nutrients into your body in an easy-to-absorb (and delicious) format. Fresh juices are satisfying, fill you up, give you energy, and improve your metabolism. Fresh juices are among the most nutrient-dense foods you can put into your body.

6. **Plant-based diet.** I am not saying you "have to" become a vegan or even a vegetarian in order to be optimally healthy. As we have seen, some animal foods are very nutrient-dense for

important nutrients. Eggs, for example are a great source of sulfur-containing amino acids and protein. But pretty much all food scientists and nutritionists today agree that an optimal diet is one that is based *primarily* on a diverse foundation of plant foods. If you choose to eat animal products, it might be best to eat them more sparingly, and make sure you choose organic and humanely raised sources.

7. **Less salt.** Salt (sodium) is certainly necessary- in very small quantities, which you can likely get from a diverse, plant-based diet. But the unnaturally large quantities that most Americans are accustomed to can have an aging, drying effect on the skin and other tissues.

8. **Cut out fried foods.** Yes, they taste great. We all love crispy, salty, fried foods. But they are absolutely not your friend if you are serious about enhancing and retaining your looks. Fried oils contain damaged, oxidized fats that are known to accelerate aging and muck with your metabolism. They may taste great- but the reality is that they are not doing your health or looks any favors.

9. **Fit in the *right* fats.** Blind "fat phobia" is unnecessary. Fats can certainly be bad (see # 8, above) but they can also be wonderfully helpful. It is all about the right fats- and distinguishing good from bad. Fresh flax oil, coconut oil, hemp oil, some fish oils and a couple others are great; fried, hydrogenated, refined oils are definitely bad for you. Avoid cottonseed oils, canola oil, corn, soybean, and peanut oils.

10. **Consider cruelty-free foods.** This is another aspect of our saying, "you are what you eat". A big part of beauty in the eyes of beholders is simply, being kind. Nice people are universally considered as more attractive. It is certainly true that throughout history people have been generally more attracted to

people who are more relaxed, gentle, and peaceful. It is a hard and sobering truth that the animal "industry" treats animals that are raised for food as mere commodities-not as sensitive living beings with feelings- and they are often treated quite horribly.

Most of these animals have inconceivably difficult lives filled with suffering and misery. Aside from being deprived of the ability to fulfill their most basic instincts, poor, unnatural diets, crowded, dirty living conditions, rampant disease, and fear and confusion characterize the life and deaths of these creatures.

This is all now very well documented and an awareness of this is something to consider as part of eating consciously. Most people are still only dimly aware of the truth of this, and many more choose to ignore the unpleasantness of this side of food production in our modern world. To be honest, this is the really "ugly side" of agribusiness in the world today. I fully acknowledge that this is not at all pleasant to think about, but I think it is very important, and is an unavoidable aspect of "eating responsibly and consciously".

11. **Minimize refined sugar intake.** We spoke of this in the chapter on the skin and also in the chapter on aging. When sugar levels are not regulated properly, higher levels in the bloodstream can join with proteins, which result in "AGES" or altered proteins that don't function very efficiently and are associate with accelerating the aging of the skin and other tissues.

12. **Diversify your diet with "super foods".** "Super foods" are special, "best of the best" most nutrient-dense foods that can contribute extra doses of specific nutrients, and in many cases, unusual nutritional molecules that may offer extra benefits. A few examples include sea vegetables, nutritional yeast, spirulina

and chlorella, bee pollen, green tea, sprouts, turmeric and certain spices, and others.

Supplements

Although diet is the foundation of health- and of the *Beautiful from Within* program, supplements also play a significant- and sometimes crucial- role in supporting challenged, stressed, or vulnerable tissues. In the chapters on skin, hair, and nails I discuss the various specific nutrients that can be useful in building healthier, skin, hair, and nails. Here is a brief summary:

- **SKIN-** essential fatty acids, vitamin C, zinc, silica, copper, MSM
- **HAIR-** sulfur amino acids (cysteine, methionine), silica, B1, biotin, essential fatty acids, zinc, copper
- **NAILS-** sulfur amino acids, silica, protein, trace minerals, MSM, magnesium

Exercise

Exercise regularly. This is probably a "no brainer" but still needs to be repeated. Exercise helps the blood carry oxygen deep into tissues and also helps it remove waste molecules and toxins. Exercise also helps stimulate and tone up the metabolism on a cellular level. And of course, exercise can assist in lowering stress hormones and increase endorphins which elevate mood. Everything from yoga to Pilates to rock climbing to kayaking counts!

Quality Time

Relaxation and down time. Quality time means finding time to do less. Instead of feeling rushed and caught in the trap of compulsively "doing" all the time, a "beautiful life" means one of balance. Being able to balance the tasks and goals we set for ourselves with quality quiet moments to relax is very important. It can be too easy to forget that life is what is happening to us *now*. A beautiful life is a balanced life filled with quality moments. When we take things too seriously we might find that the stress we are constantly experiencing can take its toll on us. Think beautiful thoughts- you are what you think!

Being beautiful means living beautifully. Give to your community, to a charity, to a cause you believe in. You can make the world a more beautiful place just by being here and doing something positive.

Smile!

Laugh!

Be grateful!

Spend time in nature!

Remember to honor yourself.

You deserve to be happy, successful, and fulfilled!

Love yourself !!

You are beautiful- inside and out !!

Appendix

Celebrating Exceptional Foods

Instead of seeing (bad) food as the problem, it is much better to see food—good food— as the solution. Since food is the central focus of a truly healthy dietary lifestyle it makes sense to celebrate delicious and satisfying foods by acknowledging and honoring them for their exceptional ability to support, nourish, and delight. Recognizing and celebrating exceptional foods alters your relationship with food in fundamental and profound ways, and is an important stepping-stone toward reconnecting with the fun of food. Whether discussing ripe luscious blueberries (which recent research has shown can actually reverse signs of aging in test animals), rich dark chocolate, liquid golden flax oil, succulent sushi, rich buffalo steaks, or a myriad of other nutrient-dense foods, the appreciation of such food marks an important step in the journey of people's ability to nourish themselves.

Most diet books today focus on the negative. Food is too often portrayed as the enemy, or as a "problem" to be solved. The society we live in seems to have developed an adversarial relationship with food. According to many diet experts, food makes you fat, zaps your energy, clogs your arteries, and gives you allergies, digestive problems, and headaches.

Yet what about the other side of the coin? Food also nourishes you, keeps you alive, and gives you great satisfaction and culinary pleasure. Food also brings people together, and provides a focal point as well as a cultural identity; it links countless generations of people who, in their time, also farmed, cooked, ate, and loved.

Creating an enemy out of one of the most central and basic aspects of life is crazy, yet the current dietary landscape is so out of balance that it makes this unprecedented negative relationship with food seem normal. Fortunately, there is a better and far healthier way to relate to food.

When you give up trying to eat in unnatural ways, you can begin to relax, reexamine your relationship with food, and start cultivating a healthy relationship with genuinely good food. Celebrating the goodness of good food is not difficult because it is actually quite natural. Embracing the ancient awareness that food should nourish, support, and strengthen can come as a refreshing surprise. It is actually a relief to discover that you can *appreciate* truly good food, instead of dreading it.

Celebrating good food is natural and normal. Fearing it as something dangerous is unnatural and, historically speaking, unprecedented. It is also unnecessary. Of course, you need to be aware of which foods to avoid, especially these days, but you also need to balance that awareness with an adequate knowledge of the many safe, healthy, and desirable foods available to you. Once you make this basic distinction, you can safely embark on a lifetime journey of healthy eating.

Wonderfully delicious, nutrient-dense foods are easy to incorporate into your diet. Celebrating these foods simply means appreciating them for what they are. Cinnamon not only tastes wonderful, but helps to metabolize and regulate blood sugar. Olive oil helps keep arteries pliable and open. Luscious blueberries and other berries help keep nervous systems strong and youthful because they contribute an important class of anti-oxidants. Seaweeds offer a storehouse of trace minerals from the world's oceans. Healthful teas give a myriad of plant-based molecules, and nuts and seeds give essential oils, protein, and other important compounds. Cocoa solids, present in dark chocolate, contain potent flavonoid antioxidants, while organic eggs and healthy meats give amino acids, fats, iron, zinc, and other vital nutrients.

It is important to like food. While working throughout the years as a nutritional consultant, coach, and doctor, I have been amazed by the many people who have expressed fear about food. Often, shame or embarrassment is mixed with their fear, a sad, unnecessary state of affairs. Yet, I have also witnessed people's ability to heal these feelings and come to a healthy appreciation of food and its place in their lives. I have seen the joy and relief that accompanies the healing of such a fractured relationship with diet.

Celebrating food is the heart of cultivating a healthy relationship with it. As with people, each food is unique, individual. At its best, a good meal should be able to shock us with its freshness, boldness, or even its simplicity. Nutrient-dense meals can be elaborate or simple, humble, and wholesome, or complex and exotic. The piquant spiciness of a perfect pomegranate, the satisfying texture and crunch of fresh walnut meat, a perfectly balanced salad, or the shape and fragrance of a piece of seaweed in a soup or stir-fry engages your senses, alerting you to the satisfaction and excitement good nourishment can accomplish.

Many people seem to find reassurance in the consistency and predictability of food purchased from chains, big-name brands, and fast-food outlets. I, however, find boredom in boxes. Although nutrient-dense foods can be obtained from commercial outlets, restaurants, and name-brand companies, the celebration of food I am referring to is more concerned with an appreciation for the individual elements so often missed when food comes in a pre-packaged or pre-made form. It is the beauty of an individual carrot, the freshness of a bright red pepper or the crispness of a bunch of fresh spinach that can reconnect you in an instant with the bounty and goodness of the earth.

Food should never be taken for granted. Thankfully, we do not have to worry about the availability of food the way our ancestors might have. Like many people, you may not be directly involved in growing, raising, hunting, or foraging for your food.

But, does this mean it is all right to undervalue it? I believe that this lack of appreciation for food is the underlying cultural eating disorder of our time, and may be partly responsible for many of the other neurotic or maladaptive attitudes toward food that are so pervasive in society today.

Celebrating good food really means trusting it. It also means trusting yourself and your innate ability to sort out what is good, and not good, for you. Trusting yourself with food also means you can begin to relax and enjoy it in a more guilt-free way. For some, this is truly difficult because the thought of food can carry a charge that makes many people deeply uncomfortable. Issues of worthiness, or body image, are feelings that can signify a deep lack of trust in food, in ourselves, and in the world itself. As a result of this relationship with food, many develop a deep ambivalence toward the ways in which they get nourished.

Organic vs. Non-Organic?

A lot of folks have the same question when they think about the transition to a more and more nutrient-dense diet. "Do I have to buy everything organic?" This is a very sensible and reasonable question!

Some foods matter more than others in terms of the importance of buying organic. If you are on a limited budget than obviously it is very important to monitor your grocery budget carefully- which probably means you will not be purchasing all organic items. Fortunately it is not necessary to be 100% organic. A few tips and suggestions might make your shopping decisions a bit simpler. Here are my top suggestions:

Certain foods are grown or raised with higher levels of pesticides, etc. than others. Those are the foods where I personally will only buy organic.

Some of the foods that are most important to purchase organically are potatoes, mushrooms, citrus fruit, grapes and raisins, pineapples and a lot of soft fruits, including melons and strawberries. This is because these crops in particular are known to be heavily sprayed. Corn is also important to buy organically because virtually all of the non-organic corn in this country is now GMO. In fact, corn, sugar beets and soy are the main GMO foods today but there are many others and their numbers are growing.

The animal industry is especially bad-and therefore all animal products need to be organic- including all milk, ice cream, yogurt, and cheese! This is because of the widespread use of chemicals including antibiotics and estrogenic hormones and because of the horrendous conditions the animals tend to be raised in. Both of these factors lead to stress, disease, and suffering on an unprecedented scale. Please do not support such practices – remember, you are what you eat! This goes for all meat- poultry, pork, and beef as well as dairy and eggs. And remember, even organically raised animals can suffer horribly. If possible, try and know where your food comes from- especially your meat and animal products.

Knowledge is power, so please realize you can do your part to help the animals and responsible farmers with your purchasing dollars. You can make a difference in your own life as well as in the lives of others if you vote with your dollars wisely!

A Nutrient-Dense Superstar Checklist:

Vegetables: Almost all vegetables are moderately to highly nutrient-dense- especially when organic and raw or lightly cooked

Fruits: Blueberries, raspberries, (all berries, really), apples, bananas, citrus, kiwi, mango, pomegranates, organic pineapple...basically all fruits, esp. when organic

Oils: Coconut oil, flax seed oil, cod liver oil, wheat germ oil, hemp oil, organic grass-fed butter, extra virgin olive oil

Carbohydrates: Blackstrap molasses, brown rice, millet, quinoa, organic baked or boiled (not fried!) potatoes (when the skin is left on), yams, raw honey

Proteins: (note: all animal products must be organic to eliminate hormones, antibiotics, and other metabolic toxins) Eggs, elk, lamb, buffalo, wild caught seafood (not farmed), some sushi, any organic meats, liver, unpasteurized cheeses and yogurt, almonds, sunflower seeds, walnuts, pine nuts, sesame seeds, peanuts, tempeh, beans, lentils, peas, brown rice, millet, quinoa.

Miscellaneous: Nutritional yeast, sea weeds, miso, bee pollen, spirulina, chlorella, nuts and nut butters, many spices and herbs, teas, sprouted grains and seeds, dark chocolate (small amounts).

The Worst Foods for Your Metabolism:

- **Alcohol**
- **Aspartame** (NutraSweet™)
- **Bad oils:** (commercial cooking oils that are non-refrigerated, including corn oil, soybean oil, canola oil, peanut oil, and cottonseed oil.)
- **Fried foods** (chips, fries, chicken...)
- **GMO corn, soy, sugar** (these are the biggest but there are many others)
- **High Fructose Corn Syrup**
- **Hormone-containing animal products** (i.e. any non-organic: eggs, chicken, milk, cheese, pork, beef)
- **Monosodium Glutamate (MSG)**
- **Partially-Hydrogenated oils, fats, shortenings and margarines**
- **White flour** (and virtually all baked goods)
- **White sugar**

Greatest Foods for Your Metabolism!

- Apples
- Beans, legumes, lentils
- Bee Pollen
- Berries- fresh or frozen
- Brown rice
- Buffalo meat, liver
- Cayenne powder
- Coconut oil
- Coconut milk
- Coconut water
- Eggs (must be organic and free range)
- Flax oil
- Fresh fruits (apples, berries, kiwis, melons, mango, pineapple, etc)
- Fresh Goat's milk
- Fresh Greens (lettuces, baby spinach, arugula, kale, etc)
- Fresh Juice (carrot, veggie blends, fruit blends, wheatgrass)
- Fresh Veggies
- Garlic

- **Ginger root**
- **Green tea**
- **Jalapenos and other hot peppers**
- **Kombucha**
- **Lemons**
- **Millet**
- **Nutritional Yeast**
- **Nuts, seeds** (preferably raw, unroasted), nut butters
- **Onions** (yellow and red)
- **Quinoa**
- **Radishes**
- **Salsa** (fresh)
- **Sauerkraut** (fresh, "live")
- **Seaweeds** (e.g. kelp, dulse, many others)
- **Shiitake mushrooms**
- **Spirulina** (and Chlorella)
- **Sprouts** (alfalfa, broccoli, mung, radish, sunflower
- **Squash** (winter and summer)
- **Umeboshi Plum vinegar**
- **Wild Oceanic fish**
- **Yogurt** (unsweetened, made from raw milk)
- **Honorable mention:** (small quantities) dark chocolate, red wine, microbrew beer

Joys of Juicing

Juicing is one of the very best ways to get concentrated nutrients in a delicious convenient form. A good juicer will extract the juice - the "life blood" of fruits and vegetables so your body can quickly absorb the nutrients. Fresh juice is full of the plant's enzymes- small molecules that are only found in "live" or "raw" (i.e. uncooked) foods. This understanding is one of the main principles behind the philosophy of eating a "live" or "raw" food diet. A good juicer is one of the few pieces of "special" equipment needed if you truly want to follow a nutrient-dense lifestyle. Juicing is easy, and can make a big difference to your sense of well-being if you incorporate it into your eating lifestyle on a regular basis. Carrots, celery, beets, ginger and cucumbers are some of the easy, commonly used vegetables along with leafy greens such as kale and spinach. Fruit is easily juiced as well and provides enjoyable, refreshing concentrated nutrition by the glassful. If you like, throw some of the pulp (fiber) back in to get additional benefits. The leftover pulp also makes great compost for your garden!

Basic Juice Recipe

Here is my basic juice recipe:
3-6 carrots (it all depends upon the size of the carrots)
1-2 stalks of celery
½ cucumber
½ apple
¼ lemon
a small piece of fresh ginger root
¼ fresh beet root

Change the proportions and ingredients depending upon your taste buds, produce availability, etc.

Nutrient-Dense Salad Dressings

Salads are a really important part of a successful nutrient-dense eating plan and an appropriately delicious and nutritious dressing is the perfect complement- both taste-wise as well as from a nutritional point of view. The following recipes will show you how to make your own fresh and delicious dressings that are far tastier and healthier than anything you can buy in a bottle. Once you find a version that you love, you will want to make a large batch and store it in your fridge. Keep some on hand in the refrigerator at work, or find a handy small bottle that you can put in your pocket or handbag when you go to a restaurant so you can have a really healthy salad away from home. These also are great for dipping vegetables!

Umeboshi Plum Vinegar

Umeboshi plums are a traditional Japanese food that is reputed to have strong health- supporting effects. These are small plums that are aged in a brine solution and allowed to naturally ferment. The soft moist salted plums are eaten medicinally as they are considered very alkaline in the macrobiotic tradition. They are also made into a paste which is also used as a delicious condiment. Umeboshi paste and vinegar are very strongly salty, so a little goes a long way! Leaves of the shiso plant are used in the preparation process which gives the plums, paste, and vinegar a beautiful rosy or purplish hue. The plum vinegar is much more salty and is more tart than it is vinegary, and has a fresh, clean, crisp "bright" taste that makes it perfect in salad dressings and as a condiment or flavoring for waking up many dishes.

Salad Dressing #1

The most basic dressing has just two ingredients. But as you will see, it is easy to start adding to this base. Surprisingly delicious! Ingredients: fresh flax oil, umeboshi plum vinegar.

Use just enough flax oil to coat the leaves of the lettuce and other vegetables, and put in a light splash or so of the vinegar and toss. Umeboshi is a light, tart, salty vinegar that gives a bright taste to things. It goes very well with good quality flax oil. Don't overdo the umeboshi- it is quite salty and a little goes a long way. Fresh flax oil (which should always be refrigerated) is a bit stronger tasting compared with ordinary, refined conventional oils so don't overdo it either!

Salad Dressing #2

This one is more complex than #1, but uses the same flax oil/umeboshi vinegar combination as a starting point. In a bottle or jar add: 2-4 oz flax oil, 1-3 Tbsp. umeboshi plum vinegar, 6-8 oz. extra virgin olive oil, a squeeze of lemon juice, ½ tsp powdered kelp or dulse, squirt of organic mustard, dollop of wasabi mayonnaise or vegan substitute. Blend or shake vigorously. Makes approx. 12 oz. of simply awesome dressing! Caution: start slowly with the umeboshi and add a little at a time until you get the right flavor. Don't overdo it!

Salad Dressing #3

Here is another variation that is simply delicious! In a bottle or jar combine:
4 oz. flax oil, 6-8 oz extra virgin olive oil, 1-2 Tbsp. umeboshi vinegar, 1 Tbsp. almond butter, 1 Tbsp. nutritional yeast flakes. Mix or shake vigorously!

Salad Dressing #4

Tahini-lemon dressing! Easy and delicious! In a bowl, bottle or jar combine: 3 Tbsp. tahini (sesame butter), ½ cup extra virgin olive oil- whisk together or blend well, add 2Tbs nutritional yeast, blend in, then add 2-3 Tbsp. fresh flax oil, a pinch of sea salt, 1 Tbsp. umeboshi plum vinegar, squeeze in a couple tsp. of fresh lemon juice. Blend or whisk all together.

Salad Dressing #5
Honey mustard yumminess! Blend together 1-2 Tbs of good raw honey with 1 Tbs of organic mustard. Blend with 3 oz flax oil and 6-8 oz extra virgin olive oil mixture. Add a dollop of almond butter and mix well. A splash of umeboshi plum vinegar will really enhance the sweet/savory marriage in this dressing
.

Salad Dressing variations: The above recipes all provide "ballpark" proportions and measurements. Rely on your own taste buds and preferences to give your dressing your own personal signature. Some great variations include blending in a ripe avocado to create a creamier "green goddess" effect. Minced or pressed garlic of course is a classic addition for many salad dressings. You can also add in a little of the juice from the olives you purchase from the deli or olive bar- briny olive water is super flavorful and adds a really nice dimension to a dressing. Black pepper is also an important addition to many dressings.

Fresh herbs are both nutrient-dense as well as delicious! Whether from the store, a farmer's market, or your own or a neighbor's garden, it's great to add some freshly diced tarragon, cilantro, mint, basil, or oregano. I also like to add some nutritional yeast to many of my dressings- this really boosts the nutritional denseness of the dressing and brings a nice subtle nutty savory-ness to the dressing. A sprinkle of powdered kelp or dulse can also provide more complexity to the finished taste profile as well as contributing trace minerals.

Eggs

Eggs are a perfect nutrient-dense food and a great way to start the day- but only if they are truly free-range and certified organic. Healthy eggs are full of good lipids, lecithin, B vitamins, vitamin A, and protein along with healthy cholesterol- an important nutrient that our nervous systems require to function optimally. Unfortunately many of us have been taught to be "afraid" of eggs- because (so we are told) the cholesterol will cause heart disease. If you prepare your eggs the way I recommend, cholesterol will be your good friend and not your enemy! We actually need cholesterol- we make our favorite hormones- progesterone, estrogen, and testosterone- out of cholesterol in addition to our anti-stress corticosteroid hormones. The key is to not damage the cholesterol – a process called oxidation-which occurs when we burn or over cook it. Excessive heat such as from frying will damage cholesterol and it is this damaged cholesterol that is bad for us. But in its healthy undamaged state cholesterol is an incredibly important nutrient. To preserve cholesterol in its "good" form, cook your eggs at a lower temperature. Instead of frying your eggs, boil them. Poaching and hard or soft-boiled eggs are a great way to enjoy them and get the benefits without the worry.

Nutrient-Dense Egg Salad
And Devilled Eggs

Egg salad can make a great snack or lunch option. Eggs are a super nutrient-dense food that provides numerous nutrients from protein, to good fats and healthy cholesterol to vitamin A to the mineral sulfur. However it is really important to get healthy "clean" eggs from certified organic, free-range hens. Commercial eggs are highly contaminated with antibiotic and hormone residues- please do <u>not</u> eat them! Here is a great way to "nutrify" ordinary egg salad and transform it into a more nutrient-dense version. Eat it by itself, by the spoonful, or on rice cakes or on gluten free or nutrient-dense bread or toast anytime of the day. This is highly nutritious and great for your metabolism so give it a go!

Note: these are very general, approximate, "ballpark" amounts- adjust the amounts by listening to your own taste buds. The important thing is the *quality* of what is used, not how much!

4-6 free range, hard boiled eggs, peeled.
2-3 Tbs fresh flax seed oil
1 tsp organic mustard
dash or two of sea salt
dash black pepper
1 Tbs nutritional yeast (optional) note: nutritional yeast
has a strong taste for some people; if you love it, use more,
if you hate it, omit it entirely!
1 celery stalk, finely diced
1 -2 Tbs of red onion, finely diced

Mix all ingredients and mash it up! The main difference between this egg salad and most ordinary ones is that we are substituting fresh flax oil for the less healthy mayonnaise that is typically used. If your egg salad is too dry, add more flax oil, or a dash of extra virgin olive oil.

Variations: mix in some chopped pitted olives and/or capers. A dash of cayenne will warm it up if you like heat. If you are adventurous, a little wasabi powder makes a delicious change of pace. Finally, a sprinkling of dark purple dulse flakes adds beautiful sparkles of color, taste, and nutrition.

Note: for devilled eggs, essentially do the same as above but slice the eggs in half length-wise. Separate the yolks and add the oil, mustard, salt, and pepper to the yolks and mash until smooth. Then fill in the egg white "boats". Sprinkle a little paprika or turmeric on top for a "traditional" look or some deep purple dulse flakes for a nice effect.

Unmatchable Matcha

One of the hottest beauty secrets is a relatively unknown beverage from Japan- one of the world's true originators of the beauty from within concept. Practically everyone today knows that green tea is considered a supremely healthy beverage. Loaded with antioxidants and a uniquely effective "anti-stress" compound, theanine, green tea consumption has been investigated by researchers for its possible ability to prevent or slow down the onset of some cancers, and for its association with longevity. What most people don't know is that the "greenest of the green" teas is a unique form called Matcha.

Matcha is tea that is specially grown under shade canopies and carefully harvested to retain the most sensitive and precious anti-aging and antioxidant constituents. As a result, high quality matcha has a vibrant, bright emerald green color that testifies to its freshness and potency. Unlike traditional teas where the leaves are steeped and then tossed away, matcha is stone ground- in fact, it is so finely powdered that it completely dissolves in hot water. In other words, when you drink matcha tea, you are consuming the whole, young, tender leaves- so you get all of the nutrients from the tea leaves.

From a "beautiful from within" standpoint, matcha is truly unmatchable. Matcha is an extremely rich source of substances known as catechin polyphenols- strong antioxidant compounds that scavenge or neutralize free-radicals that attack healthy tissues and which can cause inflammation, tissue damage, and accelerate aging. Some studies indicate that matcha may even assist in weight loss among other benefits.

Matcha is starting to become available where fine teas are sold, but it is still a relative newcomer to American shelves and is not nearly as common or easy to find as other green and black teas. I recommend matcha from reputable, certified Japanese growers and plantations. One of the very best comes from a fifth generation family-owned matcha company, called AOI. AOI offers extremely high quality matcha at great prices. They are a wonderful company based in Japan and in California. Their website is www.aoitea.com and their # is: 714-841-2716. They offer a complete line of premium matchas as well as some other fine teas. Enjoy!

e.g.

Pages 104 through 116 have been reprinted with permission from *The Nutrient-Dense Diet* (Organic Healthy Living, Inc. Publications)

Glossary

AGEs (Advanced Glycation End-products) Ages are molecules in the body that are produced from the interaction of sugars and proteins. They are found in cells and tissues that are damaged or aging.

Amino acids small molecules that usually contain nitrogen and which link together to create proteins. Some amino acids contain sulfur in place of nitrogen.

Anti-oxidants Anti-oxidants are protective nutrients that help neutralize or counteract the damage from free-radicals. Examples of antioxidant nutrients include vitamin C and vitamin E and bioflavonoids and pigments from fruits and vegetables.

Calories Calories are units of energy from food. Calories only come from carbohydrates, fats, and proteins.

Cholesterol Cholesterol is an important and essential molecule found throughout the body including our skin. Our liver manufactures it, and the body converts cholesterol into sex hormones such as progesterone, estrogens, and testosterone, and also into anti-stress hormones such as corticosteroids.

Collagen Collagen is a structural protein found throughout the body. Collagen gives our body strength, flexibility, and firmness. Vitamin C is necessary for its manufacture.

Dermis The middle layer of skin, the dermis underlies the epidermis and is responsible for much of the skin's thickness and other properties.

Empty Calories Empty calories are calories that provide energy but no nutrient value. They are the calories most commonly supplied by white flour, white sugar, and alcohol.

Epidermis What we normally think of as our "skin", the epidermis is the outermost layers of skin cells and the part of our skin that is in actual contact with our external environment.

Free Radicals Free radicals are unbalanced molecules that are usually missing an electron. Free radicals attack neighboring molecules and cells in an attempt to "rob" nearby electrons and in the process can cause chain reactions that can lead to cellular damage and tissue inflammation.

GMOs (Genetically Modified Organisms) Plants and animals that have had genes "spliced in" from other species and that are widely used by the food industry (see: S.A.D.). Common GMOs are corn, sugar beets, canola oil, soybeans, and many others. Commercial cows' milk and dairy products use GMO growth hormones.

Hydrogenated oils These are chemically altered fats and oils that create "trans-fats". These are widely used by the food industry to improve shelf life, crispness in clog arteries and lead to other health problems.
Keratin   Keratin is the main protein found in hair and nails. Keratin is a protein that contains a high percentage of sulfur in its amino acids (its building blocks).

Lipids Another word for both fats and oils.

Nutrient-Dense Nutrient-dense foods are concentrated or very good sources of nutrients such as certain vitamins, minerals, amino acids, pigments, etc. Nutrient-dense calories are calories that are accompanied by these nutrients, and are the opposite of "empty-calories". Sometimes "nutrient-dense" foods are abbreviated as "nude"foods or "NuDe" foods.

Oxidative Stress The scientific term for the damage or pressure from free-radicals.

Protein Proteins are important biological molecules assembled in the body by stringing together their building blocks, known as amino acids. Most proteins are composed mostly of amino acids that have a lot of nitrogen in them but some proteins, such as Keratin and Collagen, contain sulfur-containing amino acids.

S.A.D. (Standard American Diet) The name given to the modern diet of highly processed food, often characterized by empty calories, preservatives, GMOs, synthetic hormones, and other chemical additives

D. Lewis

Is an author, researcher, nutritionist and lecturer with a passion for helping people become healthier through nutritional awareness. He resides in southern Colorado.

docdawa@gmail.com

Graphics and Book Layout
Peter Brooks Hale

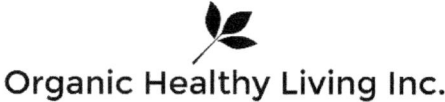

Organic Healthy Living Inc.

Publications
2015
Fort Collins, Colorado

www.ingramcontent.com/pod-product-compliance
Lightning Source LLC
Chambersburg PA
CBHW070705290526
45790CB00001B/460

* 9 7 8 1 5 0 8 5 2 6 1 0 0 *